THE
MEN'S HEALTH
GUIDE TO
INTERMITTENT
FASTING

© 2020 by Hearst Magazines, Inc.

Printed in China

Photographs by Danielle Occhiogrosso Daly and Getty Images

Book design by Laura White

Library of Congress Cataloging-in-Publication Data is on file with the publisher.

978-1-950099-40-5

4 6 8 10 9 7 5 paperback

HEARST

THE MEN'S HEALTH GUIDE TO

INTERMITTENT FASTING

From the Editors of Men's Health

Build Muscle and Torch Fat without Stressing About What You Eat

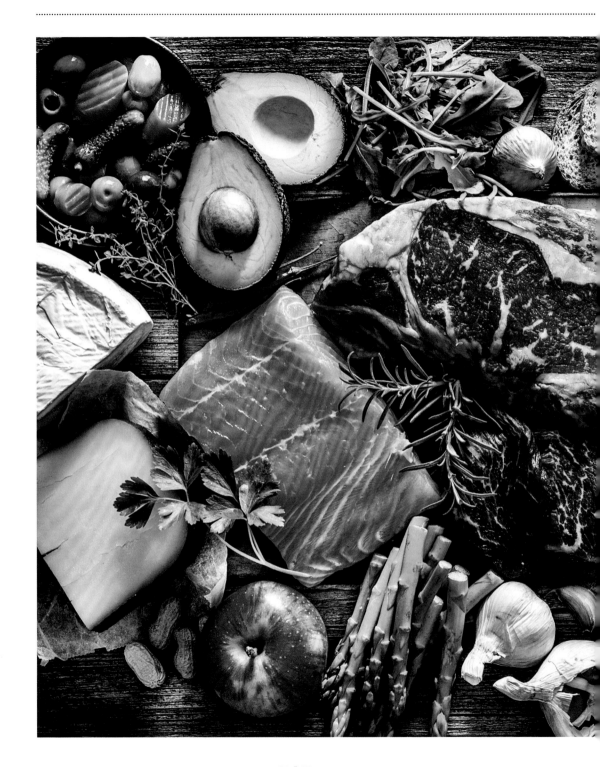

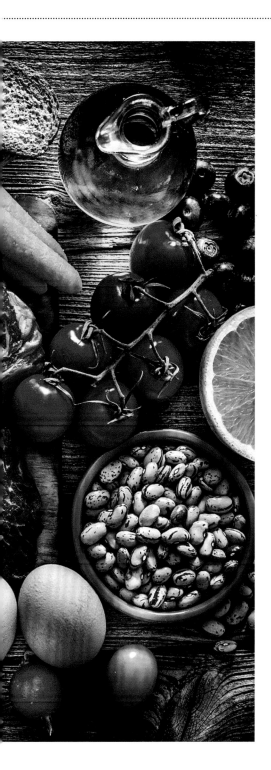

CONTENTS

EVERYTHING YOU NEED TO KNOW ABOUT INTERMITTENT FASTING

■ WHAT IS INTERMITTENT FASTING?

OKAY, WE'LL BE HONEST. Intermittent fasting is not rocket science. It's not even fifth-grade science. You might be wondering why you need a guide to tell you how to do something you do every day. But if you've ever been stuck in traffic without a snack or on the verge of eating your own laptop during a long-winded lunch meeting, you know going too long without food can mess with you. Big time. Armed with the right knowledge, however, you can use that absence of food to your physical and mental advantage.

Intermittent fasting, or IF, is just what it sounds like: the practice of periodically abstaining from eating. The idea is nothing new. In fact, humans have been partaking in periods of fasting since ancient times. What's becoming clear, however, is its powerful potential to aid in the (arguably) equally ancient quest to lose weight.

"What we previously thought—that going longer periods between meals would slow metabolism—doesn't hold weight anymore. In fact, many studies suggest that intermittent fasting may be a healthier way to eat, be a more effective approach for weight loss, and even slightly boost your metabolism," says Carolyn Williams, Ph.D., R.D.

Williams decided to try IF 2 years ago for an article she was writing on what it's like to adopt the popular diet. She admits her expectations for long-term success were low.

"One of my biggest concerns with IF was how it would affect blood glucose levels and energy. I was used to eating regularly throughout the day, so I was worried that fasting might leave me hangry and not the most pleasant mom or coworker to be around," says Williams.

Shortly after starting a 16:8 plan (in which you fast for 16 hours and consume all daily calories in an 8-hour window), Williams experienced the opposite of what she anticipated. She actually *liked* fasting. She didn't feel hungry or weak. Her energy levels were slightly higher. Her hanger? Nonexistent.

Williams found that IF kept her blood sugar levels more stable compared to when she ate more frequently during the day, and she didn't feel ravenous when it was time to break her fast. But here's the best part: she could still meet friends at a restaurant for lunch or dinner (even if said restaurant didn't have a single carb- or gluten- or *whatever-the-hell-everyone's-avoiding-these-days*-free item on the menu). She's been hooked on IF ever since.

Today's fasting techniques offer something for just about anyone. You can choose to fast every day for a certain number of hours or fast more intensely just a couple days per week. Your social feeds have probably already told you, but here it is again: people of all ages and activity levels are trying IF and dropping pounds. And as it's being studied more, research also suggests that IF can be a healthy, effective approach to weight loss and may even offer additional protection from diabetes, heart disease, and other chronic diseases.

The Science

It's about more than calories. Here's how fasting taps into your insulin and glucose levels to boost weight-loss potential.

- The carbohydrates, proteins, and fats we consume supply calories (aka energy) to the body. When digested and absorbed, carbs and protein trigger the release of insulin. Fat does not.

- Insulin is a hormone made by the pancreas that regulates blood sugar and other hormones. It's essential in helping cells break down glucose for energy.

- When we consume calories over the whole day, our glucose and insulin levels are constantly fluctuating.

- This ongoing release of insulin means that the body rarely has a need to break down fat stores for energy. Higher insulin levels have also been linked to obesity and insulin resistance.

- When we shorten our calorie-consumption window, like in a 16:8 fast, we minimize the constant release of insulin and force the body to find alternate fuels—like body fat—for energy.

While research on how IF affects humans is still limited, results are very promising. In fact, a 2017 review of existing IF studies on humans in *Annual Review of Nutrition* found that weight loss was statistically significant. The analysis also noted reductions in insulin and glucose levels in several studies, leading researchers to suggest that IF promotes weight loss and improves metabolic health, decreasing diabetes risk.

Unlike a lot of weight-loss tactics, IF doesn't require you to count calories or macros, and you don't have to track what you're eating. What matters most is *when* you eat not what. Of course, you can't eat anything on an intermittent fasting plan and lose weight. Since eating is restricted to certain times or days, it's important to eat a varied diet and choose nutrient-dense foods so you'll cover all your nutritional bases. Williams recommends doing this by focusing on whole and minimally processed foods to get these three components:

- Lean proteins (both plant- and animal-based)
- High-fiber plant foods such as fruits, vegetables (including starchy ones), and whole grains
- Healthy fat sources

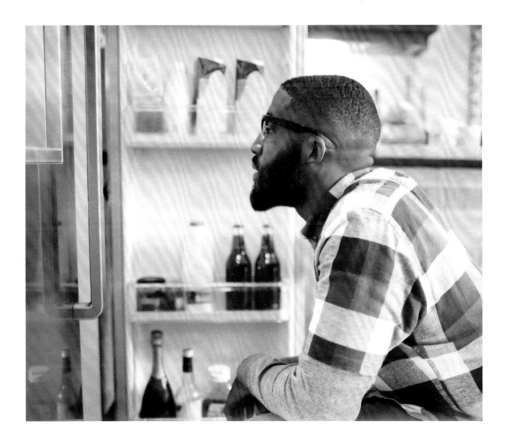

FIVE **GOOD REASONS** why you would ever consider skipping breakfast

■ We know that sometimes the only thing rousing you from bed in the morning is the prospect of a monstrously stacked bacon, egg, and cheese on a bagel. But waiting a few hours for your first meal can have a positive impact on your health. It is important to note that research into the benefits of IF is still very new, but the studies that have been conducted are promising. Fasting may help you:

ONE
DROP POUNDS

Studies have shown that both time-restricted and whole-day fasting can lead to weight loss. According to a 2018 study published in *Obesity*, IF has also been shown to help promote weight loss even if you don't cut calories from your diet. Just by changing when you eat, you can transform your body.

TWO
FOCUS MORE

Fasting adopters say that going without food allows them to do more work—and do it better—than they've ever been capable, and it's not just because they spend less time dealing with meals.

It may have something to do with adrenaline, sleep, or both. You've fully metabolized your last meal after 10 to 16 hours, depending on how much you ate. That's when your body transitions from "fed" to "fasted," releasing a symphony of hormones including testosterone and cortisol, and a host of lesser-known biochemicals that signal your body to mobilize and burn energy stores, says biochemist Trevor Kashey, Ph.D., founder of Trevor Kashey Nutrition. "Your body generates energy by burning fat, while arousing it with adrenaline, which increases your alertness and focus."

THREE
REDUCE INFLAMMATION

A 2015 study from Yale Medical School went one step further, finding that both dieting and fasting produce a compound that prevents the immune system from making a protein linked to inflammatory diseases like diabetes and atherosclerosis.

FOUR
LOWER YOUR BLOOD PRESSURE

One study published in *Cell Metabolism* in 2018 linked intermittent fasting and lower blood pressure. Researchers followed a small group of obese men with prediabetes. Some were put on a 16:8 intermittent fasting diet, while others ate over a period of 12 hours. Both groups didn't gain or lose weight. But after 5 weeks, the men in the 16:8 group significantly lowered their blood pressure and said they had decreased appetites. They weren't as hungry as they were before, even though they were fasting.

FIVE
CONTROL YOUR APPETITE

It might seem counterintuitive, but appetite control is a big benefit of fasting. A recent study in the journal *Obesity* showed that people who ate only during a 6-hour window, compared to following a normal eating schedule, felt less hungry than the control group, even though both groups ate the same amount of calories.

■ HOW TO GET STARTED

Follow these tips to start your fast on the right foot, and you'll be more likely to stick with it past week 1.

Talk to Your Doctor

Start by checking in with an expert, like your doctor or a dietitian, to make sure IF is right for you. People who have diabetes or higher caloric needs, including those who are underweight, younger than 18, or pregnant or breastfeeding, should avoid fasting, says Williams. Also, certain medications can affect how your body handles insulin and glucose, so check with your health care provider first if you have any concerns.

Know Your Options

There are several approaches to fasting. Here's a breakdown of the most common fasting schedules:

ALTERNATE-DAY FASTING entails switching from days without food restrictions and days that include one meal that provides about 25 percent of your daily calorie needs, according to Harvard Health Publications. For example, you might eat one 400-calorie meal on Monday and resume your normal diet on Tuesday.

WHOLE-DAY FASTING is also known as the 5:2 fasting schedule, which means you eat roughly 500 calories 2 days a week. The other 5 days you consume your normal calorie intake.

TIME-RESTRICTED FASTING typically follows a 16:8 format, meaning you only eat within an 8-hour window each day and the other 16 you fast. Williams suggests setting your eating window from noon to 8 p.m. so you spend a large portion of your fast sleeping and only have to skip breakfast.

Think about Your Schedule

Whether you've been following the same daily routine for years or have been known to drop everything for the right happy hour, you can fast to suit your lifestyle and still get lean in the process. A few things to consider:

ARE MOST DAYS UNPREDICTABLE? A 5:2 fasting schedule, in which you eat very minimal calories for 2 days and eat whatever you want (within moderation) the rest of the week, may work best.

DO YOU FOLLOW THE SAME ROUTINE (ALMOST) EVERY DAY? Go for a 16:8 approach, and you won't have to drastically shake up your schedule. Plus, you'll be able to eat at your regular calorie level every day.

Personalize and Prep

A little prep work will make switching to fasting easier. Based on the schedule you've chosen, think through the next few days of fasting. No matter what approach you choose, start on a busy day, suggests Williams. You'll have less time to watch the clock in anticipation of your first meal.

FOR ALTERNATE DAY OR 5:2 FASTING: Identify what days will be easiest for fasting. Williams suggests choosing days you're less likely to have conflicts, disruptions, or other obligations that might involve eating.

FOR TIME-RESTRICTED OR 16:8 FASTING: Think through what 8-hour eating window would work best for you. If you typically finish dinner at 8 p.m., you might choose to eat from noon to 8 p.m. (which means you'll fast from 8 p.m. to noon the next day).

Williams recommends starting with time-restricted fasting because it is easy to adapt to most schedules and allows for flexibility, so we'll focus on a 16:8 schedule for this guide. If this seems overwhelming, start by setting a goal to fast for 12 to 14 hours. Then, gradually increase your fasting window as you get the hang of things and feel more comfortable. While greater benefits appear to come from longer fasts, research suggests that even 12 hours of fasting can do some good.

■ SURVIVING THE SWITCH

Everyone reacts to IF differently. In the first few days, you may experience:

- ■ Mild hunger or weakness
- ■ Fatigue
- ■ Light-headedness

Williams says these side effects are fairly normal, but if they are occurring daily, you might need to shift your carb intake. Eat carb-rich foods during the first half of your eating window and avoid refined carbs and added sugar. A key part of IF is learning to listen to and interpret your body's signals, which sometimes can be due more to appetite (the desire for food) rather than true hunger (the need for food).

Williams notes that she didn't experience much hunger or weakness when starting IF. Her biggest challenge was getting past the mental hurdle of fasting.

"The idea that you're not going to eat for a certain period of time can be intimidating and overwhelming," she says. "I had to work at not letting my mind get the best of me. I also had to work at learning to listen to my body's cues, something that eating every few hours had gotten me out of the practice of doing."

After a few days of fasting, assess how you're feeling. Try another approach or decrease the time if the fasting schedule you're on doesn't feel sustainable. If at any point during the fasting process you experience more intense hunger or weakness or feel that you are jeopardizing your health, break your fast and return to your usual eating schedule, says Williams.

■ WHAT TO EAT

The goal of time-restricted fasting is not to significantly slash calories. It is to control the time period in which those calories are consumed. That means you're going to need to be vigilant about fitting a full day's worth of nutrients into your newly shrunken eating window. That may sound simple, but here's the thing: you might not even feel like eating that much because reduced appetite is a common side effect of fasting. Not gonna happen, you say? We hear you and humbly ask that you suspend your disbelief long enough to read these vital tips.

▶ **DURING A 16:8 FAST,** Williams suggests eating two large meals with two to three snacks. When planned correctly, this can provide adequate energy and nutrients for the average active male.

Meal	Calories	Make sure it includes:
MEAL 1	500–750	Lean protein Complex carbohydrates from vegetables, including starchy ones, legumes, and whole grains Other carbohydrates from fruit and/ or milk products Healthy fats
SNACKS	300–500	Fiber Protein Healthy fats
MEAL 2	500–750	Lean protein Complex carbohydrates from vegetables, including some starchy ones, and legumes Healthy fats

Pro Tip: In your hungriest moments, resist the temptation to call a grocery store rotisserie chicken "breakfast." A plate filled with a variety of foods will serve you better and decrease the chances you ever feel famished enough to consider such a thing in the first place.

Here's What Will Ruin Your Fast

The good news is you don't have to subsist solely on water and the promise of a leaner physique during your fasting window. Because there isn't a ton of research on what technically will break your fast, there is little consensus on what you can and cannot consume, says Williams. In general, stick to liquids that contain no added sugar and use this list to help you navigate everything else.

▶ **FASTING FOOD LIST**

OK	NOT OK
Black coffee on its own or with under 40 calories' worth of:	Anything with added sugar
Milk	Any solid foods
Cream	Lattes, cappuccinos, specialty coffee drinks
Stevia	Alcohol
Stevia-sweetened sugar-free syrups	Juices
Cinnamon	Sodas
Unsweetened cocoa	Kombucha
MCT oil	Gummy vitamins
Butter	
Unsweetened tea	
Naturally flavored waters	
Seltzer	
Sugar-free mints and gum	
CBD (not in gummy form)	

Why You Should Be Putting Fat in Your Coffee: Healthy fats help you feel full without breaking your fast, says Williams. That's because the calories in fat don't trigger an insulin response when consumed. Try blending 1 to 2 Tbsp of fat (like MCT oil or butter) into black coffee for a frothy, satisfying drink. Just remember to factor these added calories into your total intake for the day.

■ THE SECRET TO NEVER FEELING HANGRY

It *is* possible to go 16 hours without eating and never once want to bite someone's head off during your commute. Follow these tips from Williams so you don't spend your entire fast dreaming of donuts:

During Your Eating Window

The best way to make sure you never feel hangry when fasting is to get the most out of your eating window. You don't need to eat a ton of

SIX TRICKS for breaking your after-dinner snacking habit

■ If you're following a noon to 8 p.m. eating window, you'll have a few hours of temptation to snack before hitting the hay. Use these tips for fighting even the most aggressive case of munchies:

ONE

BRUSH YOUR TEETH AFTER DINNER.

Just do it. Your breath will be fresh, your daily oral hygiene to-dos will be complete, and suddenly you won't be thinking about food. Brushing your teeth after dinner can help signal to your brain that the eating phase of your day is over, says Williams.

TWO

FIND AN ACTIVITY FOR YOUR MIND.

Dive into a new book or Netflix series, work on a crossword or Sudoku puzzle, or plan your next vacation online. Finding a focus to keep your mind busy means less time to question your ability to fast—or count the hours until you eat again.

THREE

CHANGE YOUR NIGHTLY ROUTINE.

Routines often become habit. Dinner. Couch. TV. Bag of super-processed cheesy somethings. Just doing one thing differently may help break the pattern. Try going for a walk, calling a friend, or pouring a hot mug of tea after dinner. When you replace the eating part of your routine with something else, you're less likely to feel like you're missing out on what you'd normally be doing.

FOUR

KEEP SOME "SAFE" OPTIONS ON HAND.

There may be nights when you just need something. Decaf coffee, herbal teas, and flavored waters are in no way a replacement for your favorite nightcap, but we promise they'll knock out your craving at least temporarily.

FIVE

DON'T BRING THE TEMPTATIONS HOME.

Out of sight, out of mind. Simply keeping unhealthy food out of your home is one of the easiest ways to avoid eating it. Don't totally deprive yourself, though. Just grab a single serving of your go-to treat while out instead of bringing it home, recommends Williams.

SIX

FILL UP THE RIGHT WAY DURING THE DAY.

When you consume nutrient-dense foods that hit your calorie goals throughout the day, you'll feel energized and satisfied even at the end of your fast.

calories, just the right ones. It's also important to get adequate protein in combination with fiber-rich carbohydrates and some healthy fat at every meal and snack.

MEMORIZE THIS FORMULA

The right balance of protein, carbs, and fat will fight hunger for hours. Williams advises eating at the lower end of the Dietary Guideline recommendations for carbohydrates and suggests this macronutrient breakdown:

30% PROTEIN + 45% CARBOHYDRATE + 25% FAT

▶ Here's how that figures into the meal and snack recommendations on p. 14:

	Protein	Carbs	Fat
500-cal meal	38 g	58 g	14 g
750-cal meal	56 g	84 g	21 g
300-cal snack	23 g	34 g	8 g
500-cal snack	38 g	58 g	14 g

KEEP CARBS IN CHECK

If you eat too many refined carbs, such as those in white bread, cookies, and chips, during your eating window, your stomach's bound to grumble all night. Refined carbs cause your blood sugar to spike then plummet. Low blood sugar signals to your body that you need food, making you feel hungry even if you just ate. Get your carbs from whole grains, beans, starchy vegetables, and fruits instead, says Williams. If you do eat refined carbs or foods with added sugars, eat them earlier in your eating window so your blood glucose can rebalance itself well before your fast starts.

DON'T OVERDO IT ON SHAKES

Protein shakes can be a great way to supplement your diet, but they don't always fill you up the same way good old-fashioned solid food does. Liquids travel more quickly through your stomach than solid food. Plus, blending foods pulverizes their fibers, so your body breaks them down faster. Also, watch out for added sugars in those shakes and smoothies. They can also shoot blood sugar way up and then way down.

During Your Fasting Window

FEED YOUR MIND

Mentally stimulating activities will help take your mind off your favorite binge-watching snack. Read a book or listen to a podcast. Just avoid any food-focused content. Simply looking at or thinking about food can trick your body into thinking it's hungry by releasing gastric acid into your stomach, says Williams.

DRINK UP

When you can't distract yourself from the thought of food, have something to drink. Your body easily confuses hunger for thirst, so a tall glass of water might just do the trick. In addition to water, you can have plain iced or hot tea and coffee. Keep a variety of flavored options on hand to mix things up or try infusing your water with fruit, herbs, or vegetable slices. Low-calorie beverages that have 10 calories or less are okay on occasion, but be aware that some artificial sweeteners in these drinks can affect blood sugar (and thus insulin) slightly. Try to find options sweetened with stevia or monk fruit, as these appear to have less potential to affect glucose levels.

GET YOUR SLEEP

Lack of sleep may disrupt appetite-regulating hormones, ultimately increasing hunger, according to a 2016 report by the American Heart Association. Ghrelin, a hormone that stimulates hunger, increases when you're sleep-deprived. Leptin, the hormone that signals satiety, decreases. Williams recommends getting at least 7 hours per night to help keep hunger hormones in check.

FIVE THINGS TO KNOW about working out while fasting

■ You can still pack on muscle—but your routine might not be quite the same.

ONE
YOU CAN EXERCISE WHILE FASTING.

The short answer is yes, says Jonathan Poyourow, R.D., C.S.C.S., a sports dietitian, professional chef, and associate professor of nutrition at Johnson & Wales University. But it depends on many factors, including your age, overall health, fitness level, goals, nutrition, and lifestyle. If you're a serious athlete, IF may not allow you to properly refuel when needed, so see how your body responds and go from there.

TWO
ANY TYPE OF EXERCISE IS FINE.

But you might not be feeling up to your normal intensity. During the first few weeks of fasting, your energy levels are going to be low because your protein intake will be slightly lower than normal, says Poyourow. Do what feels right.

THREE
TIMING ISN'T THAT IMPORTANT.

You'll benefit from a solid workout no matter when you fit it in. Williams notes that the most important part is getting those workouts in regularly. You may find that your energy levels are lower during your fast and that your typical 6 a.m. gym session no longer feels right. If that's the case, try working out in the middle or end of your eating window.

If you really want to amp up your weight-loss potential, Poyourow recommends timing your workout so that it happens at the end of your fast. "Studies have shown that it takes a good 10 to 12 hours to burn up your glycogen stores and switch to mainly burning fat," he explains. "So working out at the end of your fasting period means you'll be using more of your stored fat for energy." However, if you feel weak, don't push it.

FOUR
YOU'LL STILL BUILD MUSCLE.

Research suggests IF may help you maintain lean body mass. When you lose weight, you lose both fat mass and lean body mass. You really want to maintain lean body mass, and data suggests that weight loss through IF may help to do that more so than does using traditional diet methods.

"As long as you're getting enough protein and nutrients as part of a healthy, balanced diet overall, then your muscles will be just fine," Poyourow says.

FIVE
AND WATER IS STILL EVERYTHING.

You must keep drinking water, lots of water. The common rule of thumb is that adults need at least 8 (8-ounce) cups of water daily, but many need more than that—closer to 9 cups for women and 13 for men, according to the Institute of Medicine. A heavy sweat session only increases those needs, so drink up.

YOUR TOP IF QUESTIONS ANSWERED

Why am I not losing weight?

▶ If you've been doing IF, consuming appropriate calories, and eating whole, nutrient-dense foods, you are likely losing fat and making improvements to your body. Unfortunately, these wins don't always show up on the scale. Weight can fluctuate greatly on a day-to-day basis, so the scale isn't a great indicator of short-term weight changes. Skip the daily weigh-in, says Williams. Instead, focus on how your clothes are fitting and how you feel. If you absolutely need to assign some sort of number to your progress, pick one day to weigh yourself each week, and do it at the same time every week.

I'm gaining weight. What am I doing wrong?!

▶ It might seem impossible to eat more calories in an 8-hour window than in your typical all-day graze, but it is. And you might not even realize it. So, document it all. Spend a day tracking every calorie you eat, suggests Williams. The numbers might surprise you. She also recommends making sure that you are getting adequate hydration and keeping tabs on sodium intake to help with bloating and water retention.

Where does alcohol fall into all this?

▶ Your bourbons, your beers, your home brews, and any other boozy beverage of choice are safe. We're not here to ruin your buzz, but you should know alcohol = empty calories, and it will not help you lose weight. It can make managing your blood sugar levels harder and it messes with your metabolism, says Williams. Under normal conditions, the body is fueled by glucose and fat stores, and the reliance on fat stores for energy increases toward the end of one's fasting window. But when you drink, the breakdown of alcohol takes precedence from a metabolic standpoint. Fat-burning is temporarily halted until the alcohol is fully broken down and the energy from calories consumed is used up. Stick to one or two drinks, and always down 'em with a healthy meal.

Can I combine this with other diets, like keto or paleo?

▶ Yes. But do yourself a favor and focus just on fasting for a few weeks before throwing anything else into the mix, says Williams. Many people pair IF with carb-cycling and alternate normal-carb and low-carb days. Keto, paleo, and Mediterranean diets are also fair game. The key is finding an approach that is sustainable for you and provides adequate nutrients.

How do I handle going out with friends during my fasting window when they're eating and drinking?

▶ This is the beauty of time-restricted IF: you can adjust your eating window. If you go out with friends and end up ordering everything off your local Chinese restaurant's menu at 11 p.m., so be it. Don't sweat it if your eating window runs a little longer than 8 hours on occasion. The fasting window is where the magic happens, so focus on getting back on track with your 16-hour fast starting from the time of your last bite of food (or drink).

If you can anticipate where your night will go, try to extend your fast a little longer than normal. For example, instead of eating your first meal at 12 p.m., try to wait until 2 p.m. so that your eating window goes until 10 p.m.

HOW TO USE THESE
RECIPES

IF YOU PLAN on practicing IF indefinitely, you're going to want an arsenal of easy, filling, flavor-packed recipes. Ahead you will find 30 brunch and dinner recipes, plus bonus keto ideas. Every meal provides the right mix of nutrients to fill you up, build muscle, and make your fasting window fly by. Follow these tips to make this plan your own:

Mix Things Up

These are ideas to get you started. Feel free to swap out the proteins, vegetables, and other ingredients to suit your tastes or add some variety. Just make sure you get a balance of protein, fiber-rich carbs, and healthy fats every time you eat.

Repeat What You Love

If you want to eat Bear-Sized PB&J's (p. 40) every day, technically you can. Just make sure you're getting a variety of nutrients in your eating window (i.e., you can't just eat PB&J's). Find a handful of meals that work best for your schedule and feel satisfying to you. Memorize them and buy in bulk.

Meal Prep When Possible

Keep healthy ingredients on hand and prep meals in advance. When the right choice is already waiting for you in the fridge, it's so much easier to stay on track (and way less tempting to order takeout).

Wait Before Adjusting Portions

It sounds crazy, but fasting can decrease your appetite, making it even harder to hit your nutritional goals in a small eating window. Keep an eye on total calories for every meal and snack. Though this is highly individualized based on your size and activity, Williams suggests that active men aim for 2 meals between 500 to 750 calories, as well as 2 to 3 snacks that are 300 to 500 calories.

If You Go Keto, Do This

Some fasting adopters find that keto makes IF easier. Williams attributes this to the diet's two main guidelines: high fat = increased satiety and low carb = fewer blood sugar spikes. Wait a few weeks to add keto. Then, build a meal plan that is packed with low-carb veggies to ensure you get adequate nutrients.

Snack Wisely

Smart snack combos help you sneak in needed nutrients, but will also keep you energized and satisfied until your next meal. Williams recommends avoiding snacks that are predominantly carbohydrates. Instead, she suggests choosing ones that combine fiber-rich carbs with a little protein and fat.

▶ **HERE ARE SOME IDEAS TO GET YOU STARTED:**

Small banana with peanut butter

Apple or pear with almond butter

Clementines with string cheese

Fresh mozzarella, cherry tomatoes, and a drizzle of EVOO and balsamic vinegar

Greek yogurt topped with berries and walnuts

Hummus and baby carrots

Oatmeal topped with nuts

Small whole-wheat turkey sandwich

Almonds and a piece of dark chocolate

Chicken and tuna salad and crackers

Toasted chickpeas or edamame

Hard-boiled egg and popcorn

Avocado toast

Guacamole, salsa, and whole-grain chips

Cheese, whole-grain crackers, and grapes

Trail mix made with nuts, dried fruit, and a little dark chocolate

Yogurt sprinkled with higher protein granola cereal

Small bowl of black bean soup or other bean and veggie-based soup

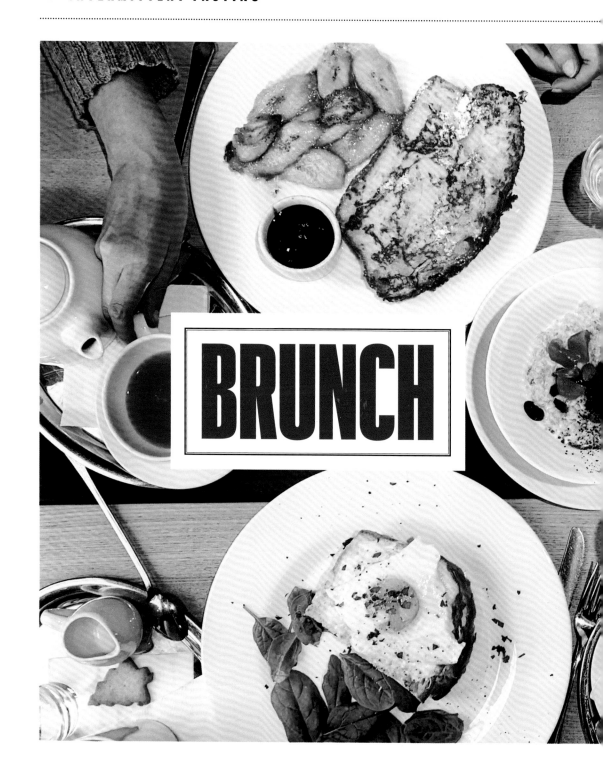

BRUNCH

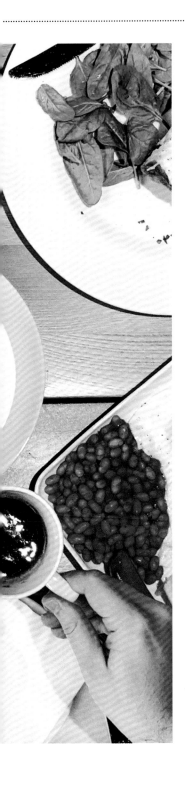

■ RECIPES

EGG SCRAMBLE
with Sweet Potatoes

TOTAL TIME: 25 MIN

WHAT YOU'LL NEED

1   (8-oz) sweet potato, diced

½   cup chopped onion

2   tsp chopped rosemary

Salt

Pepper

4   large eggs

4   large egg whites

2   Tbsp chopped chives

HOW TO MAKE IT

■ Preheat the oven to 425°F. On a baking sheet, toss the sweet potato, onion, rosemary, and salt and pepper. Spray with cooking spray and roast until tender, about 20 minutes.

■ Meanwhile, in a medium bowl, whisk together the eggs, egg whites, and a pinch of salt and pepper. Spritz a skillet with cooking spray and scramble the eggs on medium, about 5 minutes. Sprinkle with chopped chives and serve with the spuds.

MAKES 1 SERVING.

NUTRITION PER SERVING

571 calories

44 g protein

52 g carbohydrates
(9 g fiber)

20 g fat

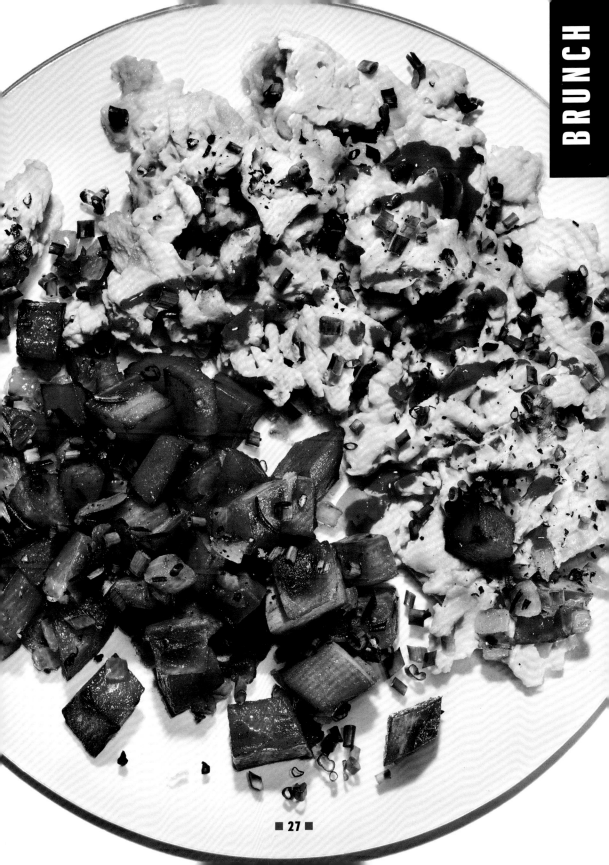

TEX-MEX BREAKFAST BURRITO

TOTAL TIME: 35 MIN

WHAT YOU'LL NEED

1¾ tomatillos, husked, rinsed, and halved

½ jalapeño, seeded and diced

3 Tbsp fresh lime juice

Cilantro, to taste

2 scallions, cut into pieces

½ tsp kosher salt

10 large eggs

1 tsp oil

1 cup canned refried beans

6 10-in. flour tortillas

2½ cups baby spinach

1 cup coarsely grated extra-sharp Cheddar

HOW TO MAKE IT

■ Heat the broiler. On a foil-lined baking sheet, arrange the tomatillos and jalapeño cut-side down. Broil until blistered, 8 to 9 minutes. Let cool, then transfer to a food processor. Add lime juice, cilantro, scallions, and ¼ tsp of the salt; pulse until combined but not smooth.

■ In a large bowl, beat the eggs with 2 Tbsp water and the remaining ¼ tsp salt. In a large nonstick skillet over medium, heat the oil. Add the eggs and cook, stirring often with a rubber spatula, to desired doneness, 2 to 3 minutes for medium-soft eggs.

■ Spread the beans on each tortilla; top with spinach, eggs, cheese, and the salsa. Fold the sides over the filling and roll from the bottom up.

■ Freeze the parchment-and-foil-wrapped burritos up to 3 weeks. To reheat, remove the foil and microwave until hot, 2 minutes per side.

MAKES 6 SERVINGS.

NUTRITION PER SERVING

505 calories

24 g protein

52 g carbohydrates (7 g fiber)

22 g fat

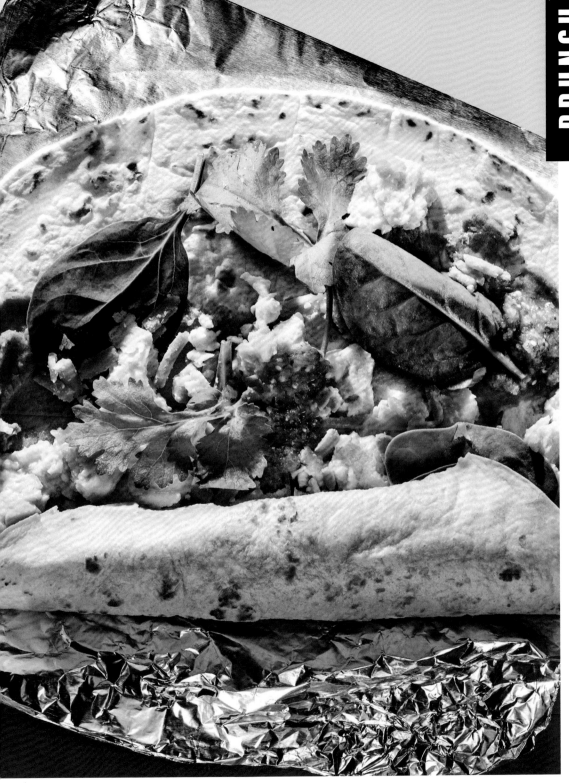

GREEK CHICKPEA WAFFLES

TOTAL TIME: 30 MIN

WHAT YOU'LL NEED

¾   cup chickpea flour

½   tsp baking soda

½   tsp salt

¾   cup plain 2% Greek yogurt

6   large eggs

Tomatoes, cucumbers, scallion, olive oil, parsley, yogurt, and lemon juice for serving (optional)

Salt and pepper

HOW TO MAKE IT

■ Preheat the oven to 200°F. Set a wire rack over a rimmed baking sheet and place in the oven. Heat a waffle iron per directions.

■ In a large bowl, whisk together the flour, baking soda, and salt. In a small bowl, whisk together the yogurt and eggs. Stir the wet ingredients into the dry ingredients.

■ Lightly coat the waffle iron with nonstick cooking spray. In batches, drop ¼ to ½ cup batter into each section of the iron and cook until golden brown, 4 to 5 minutes. Transfer the waffles to the oven and keep warm. Repeat with remaining batter.

■ Serve waffles with the savory tomato mix (left) or a drizzle of warm nut butter and berries.

MAKES 2 SERVINGS.

NUTRITION PER SERVING

412 calories

35 g protein

24 g carbohydrates (4 g fiber)

18 g fat

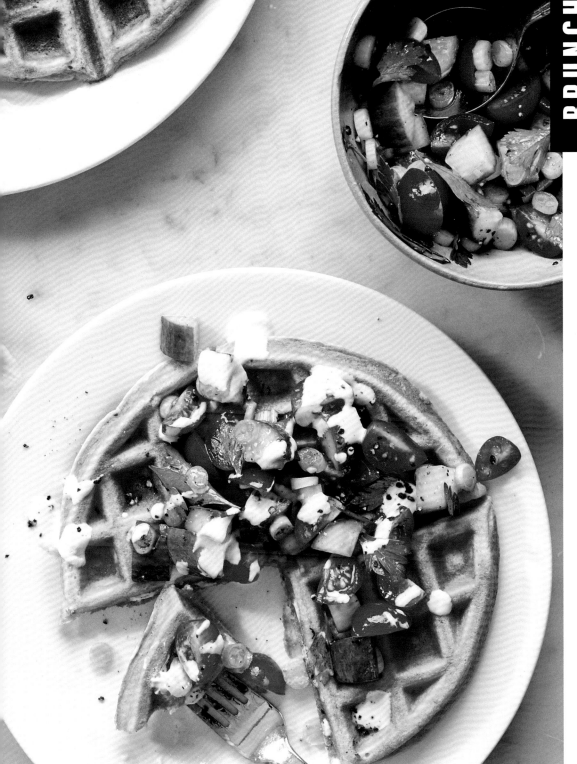

PB&J OVERNIGHT OATS

TOTAL TIME: 5 MIN (plus 8 HR for refrigeration)

WHAT YOU'LL NEED

¼ cup quick-cooking rolled oats

½ cup 2% milk

3 Tbsp creamy peanut butter

¼ cup mashed raspberries

3 Tbsp whole raspberries

HOW TO MAKE IT

■ In a medium bowl, combine oats, milk, peanut butter, and mashed raspberries. Stir until smooth. Cover and refrigerate overnight. In the morning, uncover and top with whole raspberries.

MAKES 1 SERVING.

NUTRITION PER SERVING

455 calories

20 g protein

36 g carbohydrates (9 g fiber)

28 g fat

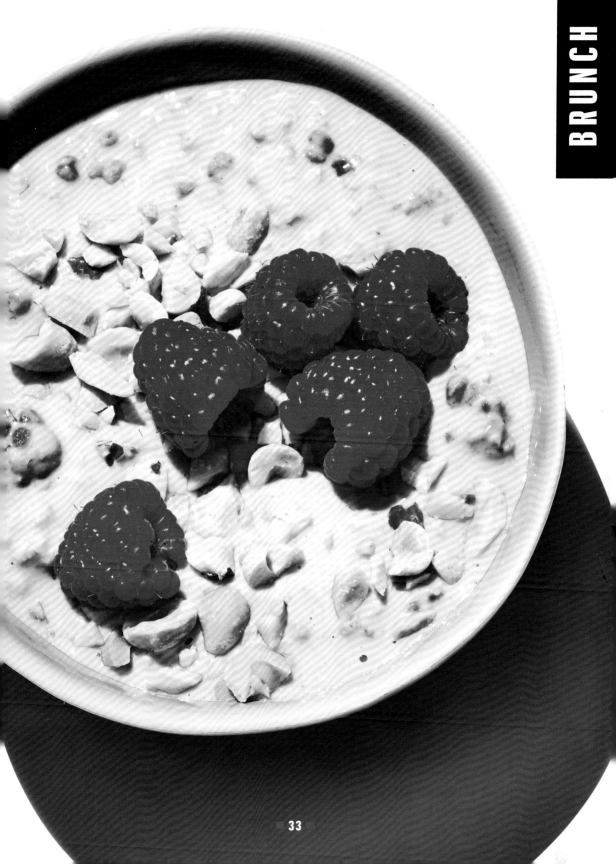

TURMERIC TOFU SCRAMBLE

TOTAL TIME: 15 MIN

WHAT YOU'LL NEED

1   portobello mushroom

3   or 4 cherry tomatoes

1   Tbsp olive oil, plus more for brushing

Salt and pepper

½   block (14-oz) firm tofu

¼   tsp ground turmeric

Pinch garlic powder

½   avocado, thinly sliced

HOW TO MAKE IT

■ Preheat the oven to 400°F. On a baking sheet, place the shroom and tomatoes and brush them with oil. Season with salt and pepper. Roast until tender, about 10 minutes.

■ Meanwhile, in a medium bowl, combine the tofu, turmeric, garlic powder, and a pinch of salt. Mash with a fork. In a large skillet over medium, heat 1 Tbsp olive oil. Add the tofu mixture and cook, stirring occasionally, until firm and egglike, about 3 minutes.

■ Plate the tofu and serve with the mushroom, tomatoes, and avocado.

MAKES 1 SERVING.

NUTRITION PER SERVING

431 calories

21 g protein

17 g carbohydrates (8 g fiber)

33 g fat

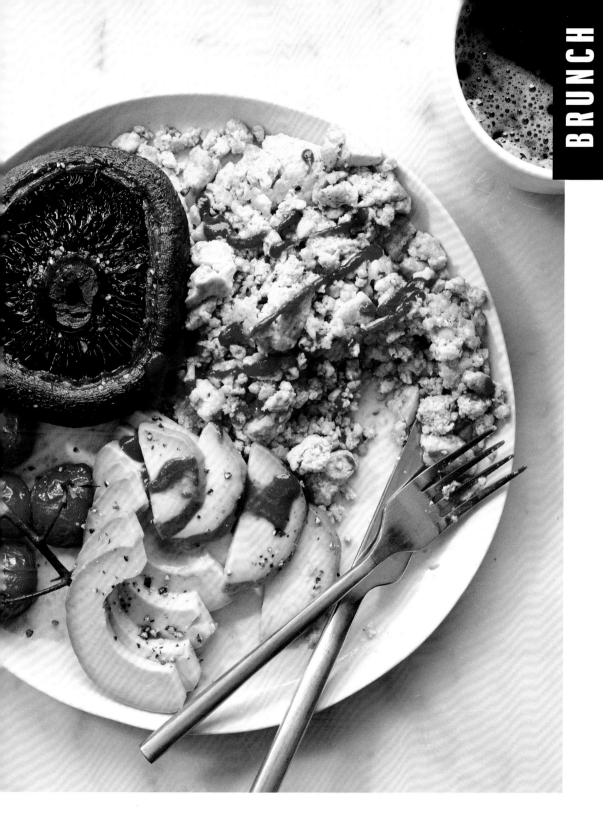

PROTEIN OATS

TOTAL TIME: 5 MIN

WHAT YOU'LL NEED

1 cup water

¾ cup oats

1½ scoops whey protein powder

½ cup whole milk

1 packet (1 g) stevia or other sugar alternative

1 tsp ground cinnamon

1 banana, sliced (optional)

HOW TO MAKE IT

■ In a microwaveable bowl, combine the water and oats. Microwave on high for 3½ minutes.

■ In a shaker bottle, combine the protein powder and milk. Shake to mix.

■ When the oats are ready, add the stevia and cinnamon. Stir to mix. Add the protein shake and stir again until mixed and smooth.

■ Add the sliced banana on top, or chow plain.

MAKES 1 SERVING.

NUTRITION PER SERVING

443 calories

42 g protein

52 g carbohydrates (8.5 g fiber)

9 g fat

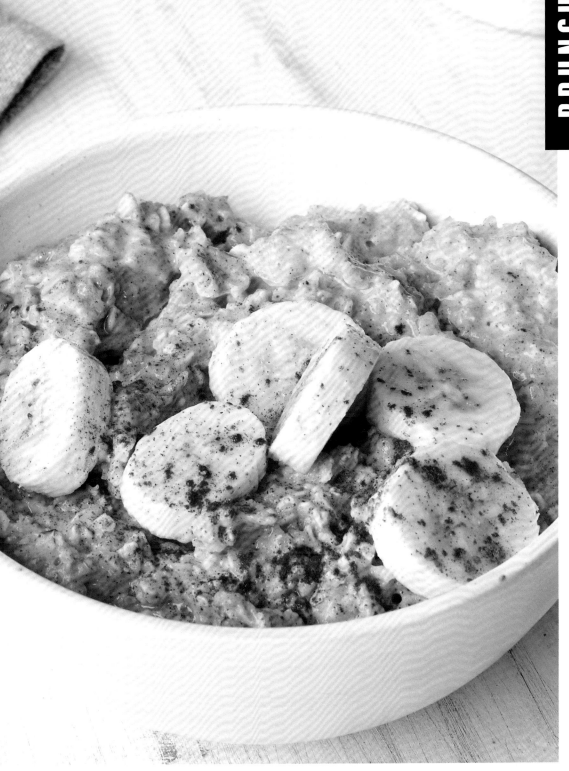

AVOCADO RICOTTA POWER TOAST

TOTAL TIME: 5 MIN

WHAT YOU'LL NEED

1   slice whole-grain bread

¼   ripe avocado, smashed

2   Tbsp ricotta

Pinch crushed red pepper flakes

Pinch flaky sea salt

HOW TO MAKE IT

■ Toast the bread. Top with avocado, ricotta, crushed red pepper flakes, and sea salt. Eat with scrambled or hard-boiled eggs, plus a serving of yogurt or fruit.

MAKES 1 SERVING.

NUTRITION PER SERVING

288 calories

10 g protein

29 g carbohydrates (10 g fiber)

17 g fat

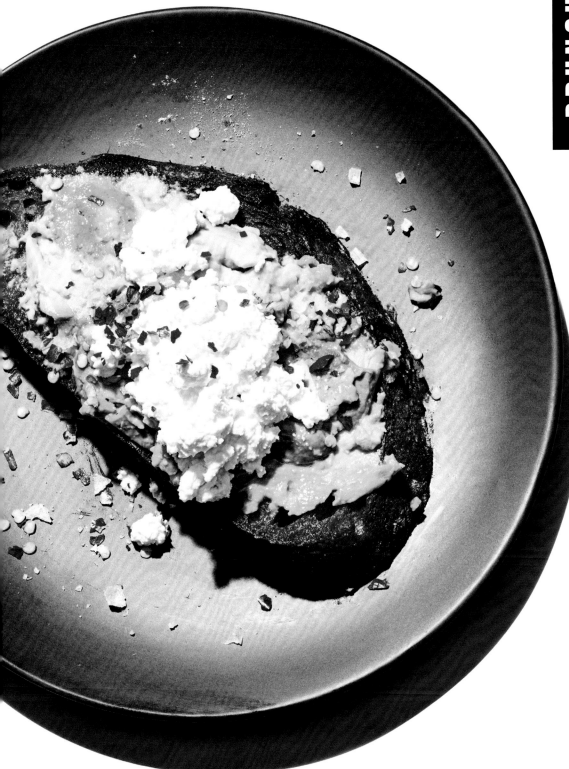

BEAR-SIZED PB&J

TOTAL TIME: 5 MIN

WHAT YOU'LL NEED

2   high-protein freezer waffles (such as Kodiak)

2   Tbsp crunchy peanut butter

⅓   cup chopped mixed strawberries and blackberries

2   Tbsp high-protein granola (such as Nature Valley)

HOW TO MAKE IT

■ Toast the waffles according to package directions. While they're warm, spread the peanut butter over one waffle. Top with the berries, granola, and the other waffle. Smush before eating.

MAKES 1 SERVING.

NUTRITION PER SERVING

682 calories

27 g protein

54 g carbohydrates (10 g fiber)

41 g fat

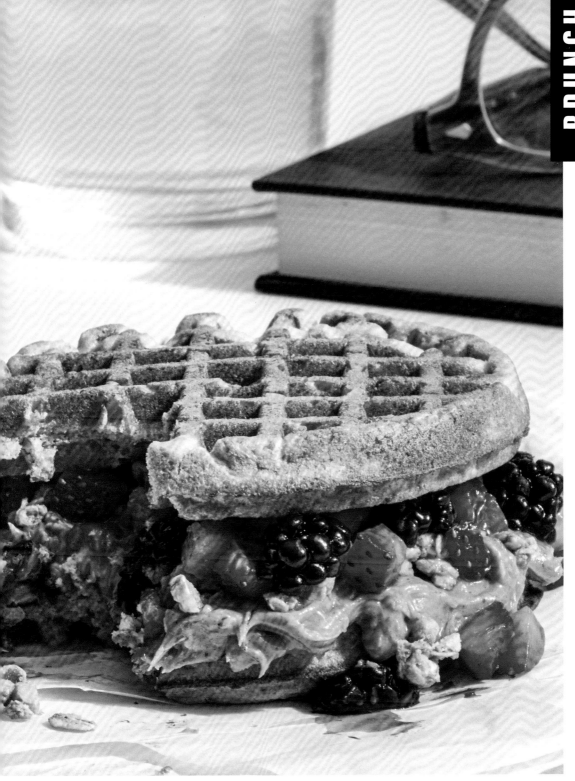

TURKISH EGG BREAKFAST

TOTAL TIME: 13 MIN

WHAT YOU'LL NEED

2 Tbsp olive oil

¾ cup diced red bell pepper

¾ cup diced eggplant

Pinch each of salt and pepper

5 large eggs, lightly beaten

¼ tsp paprika

Chopped cilantro, to taste

2 dollops plain yogurt

1 whole-wheat pita

HOW TO MAKE IT

■ In a large nonstick skillet on medium high, heat the olive oil. Add the bell pepper, eggplant, and salt and pepper. Sauté until softened, about 7 minutes.

■ Stir in the eggs, paprika, and more salt and pepper to taste. Cook, stirring often, until the eggs are softly scrambled.

■ Sprinkle with chopped cilantro and serve with a dollop of yogurt and the pita.

MAKES 2 SERVINGS.

NUTRITION PER SERVING

469 calories

25 g protein

26 g carbohydrates
(4 g fiber)

29 g fat

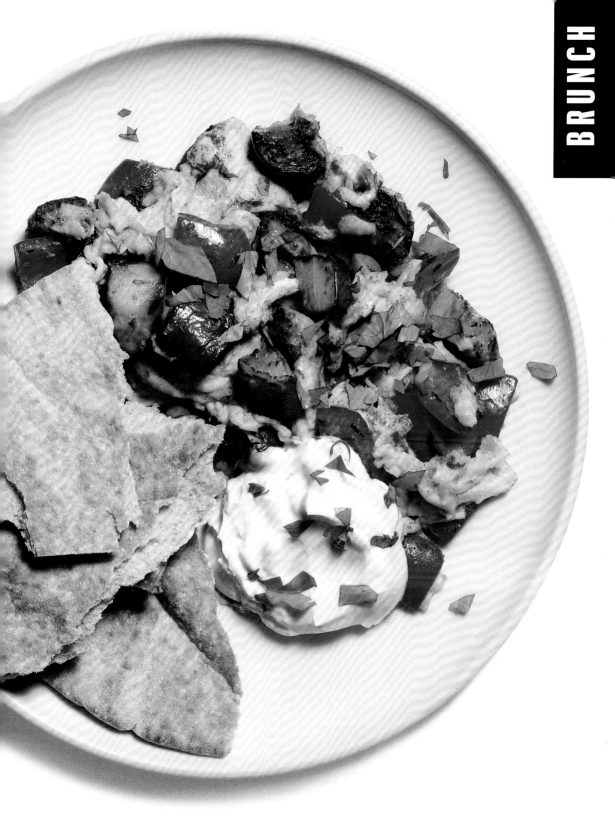

CHEESY AVOCADO OMELET

TOTAL TIME: 15 MIN

WHAT YOU'LL NEED

1	tsp olive oil
1	small red onion, finely chopped
¼	tsp kosher salt
¼	tsp pepper
6	cremini mushrooms, sliced
1	cup baby spinach
4	large eggs plus 2 egg whites
2	oz sharp Cheddar, coarsely grated
1	cup grape tomatoes, halved
¼	cup chopped fresh flat-leaf parsley
½	avocado

HOW TO MAKE IT

■ In a large nonstick skillet on medium, heat the oil. Add the onion, season with salt and pepper, and cook, stirring occasionally, for 4 minutes. Add the mushrooms and cook, stirring occasionally until just tender, 4 minutes. Stir in the spinach and cook until it begins to wilt.

■ Next, add the eggs and cook while stirring for 1 minute, then cook without stirring until the edges are brown, 2 to 3 minutes. Sprinkle with cheese and fold one half over the other to create a semicircle.

■ Toss the tomatoes with the parsley and avocado and serve spooned over the omelet. Pair with one serving of fruit or plain yogurt to make it a meal.

MAKES 2 SERVINGS.

NUTRITION PER SERVING

425 calories

30 g protein

14 g carbohydrates (5 g fiber)

30 g fat

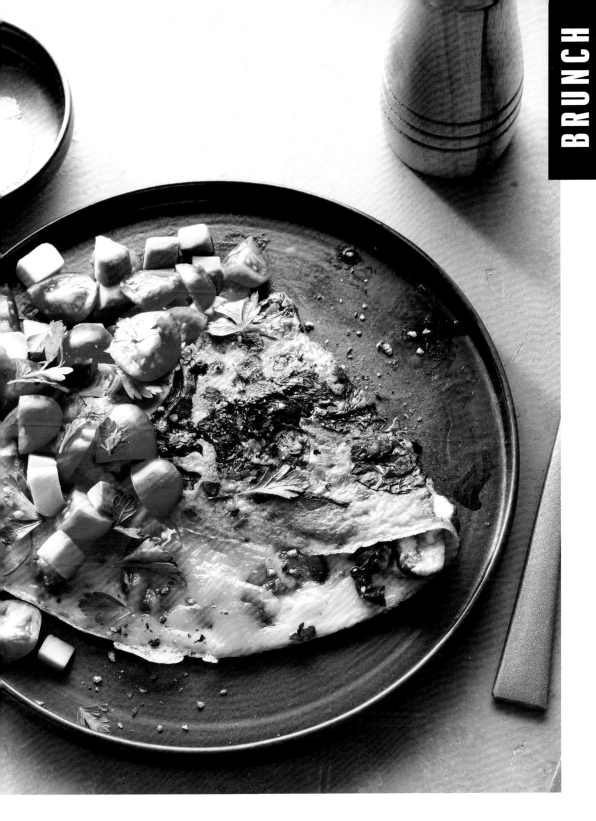

ALMOND APPLE SPICE MUFFINS

TOTAL TIME: 15 MIN

WHAT YOU'LL NEED

½   stick butter

2   cups almond meal

4   scoops vanilla protein powder

4   large eggs

1   cup unsweetened applesauce

1   Tbsp cinnamon

1   tsp allspice

1   tsp cloves

2   tsp baking powder

HOW TO MAKE IT

■ Preheat the oven to 350°F. In a small microwave-safe bowl, melt the butter in the microwave on low heat, about 30 seconds.

■ In a large bowl, thoroughly mix all the remaining ingredients with the melted butter. Spray 2 muffin tins with nonstick cooking spray or use cupcake liners.

■ Pour the mixture into the muffin tins, making sure not to overfill (about ¾ full). This should make 10 muffins.

■ Place one tray in the oven and bake for 12 minutes. Make sure not to overbake, as the muffins will become too dry. When baked, remove the first tray from the oven and bake the second muffin tin the same way.

MAKES 5 SERVINGS.

NUTRITION PER SERVING

484 calories

40 g protein

16 g carbohydrates
(5 g fiber)

31 g fat

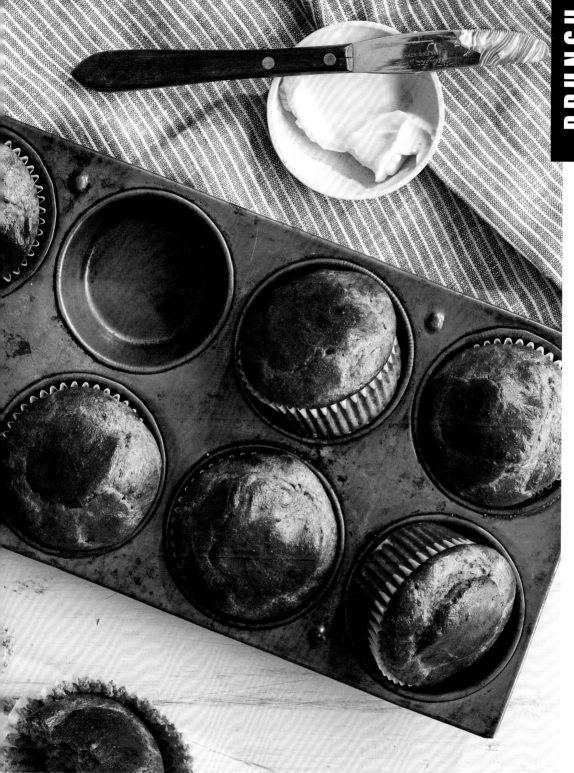

LOX, EGGS, AND ONIONS

TOTAL TIME: 13 MIN

WHAT YOU'LL NEED

1   tsp olive oil

1   medium yellow onion, finely chopped

4   oz smoked salmon, sliced into thin strips

4   large eggs or 8 egg whites

2   Tbsp whole milk

¼   tsp salt

4   Tbsp sliced scallion

4   Tbsp sliced roasted red bell peppers

HOW TO MAKE IT

■ In a large skillet coated with cooking spray over medium, heat the olive oil. Add the onion and cook for 1 minute.

■ Add the smoked salmon and cook for about 2 minutes, or until the salmon begins to turn opaque and lighter in color.

■ In a medium bowl, whisk together the eggs and milk and add to the skillet. Cook until the eggs are firm and almost dry, about 5 minutes, stirring to heat evenly.

■ Top each serving with 1 Tbsp each of the scallions and peppers. Season with salt. Eat with whole-grain toast or yogurt.

MAKES 2 SERVINGS.

NUTRITION PER SERVING

395 calories

48 g protein

8 g carbohydrates (1 g fiber)

19 g fat

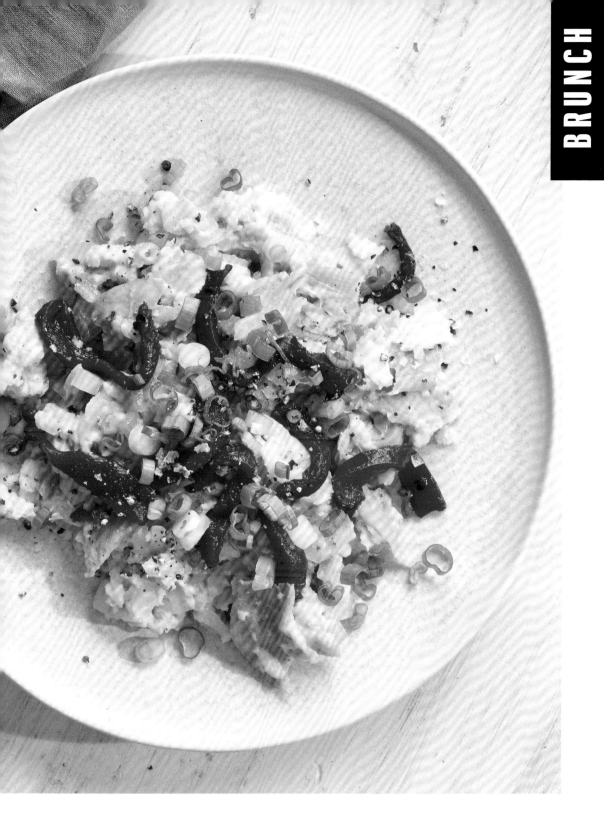

GREEK-STYLE YOGURT
with Apricots, Honey, and Crunch

TOTAL TIME: 5 MIN

WHAT YOU'LL NEED

1   cup plain Greek yogurt

5   canned apricot halves in juice, thinly sliced

4   Tbsp Grape-Nuts cereal

1   Tbsp slivered almonds

1   tsp honey

HOW TO MAKE IT

■ Spoon about half of the yogurt into a parfait glass. Top with 2 Tbsp each of the apricots and cereal. Repeat. Top each with half the almonds and honey.

MAKES 1 SERVING.

NUTRITION PER SERVING

498 calories

29 g protein

63 g carbohydrates (8 g fiber)

17 g fat

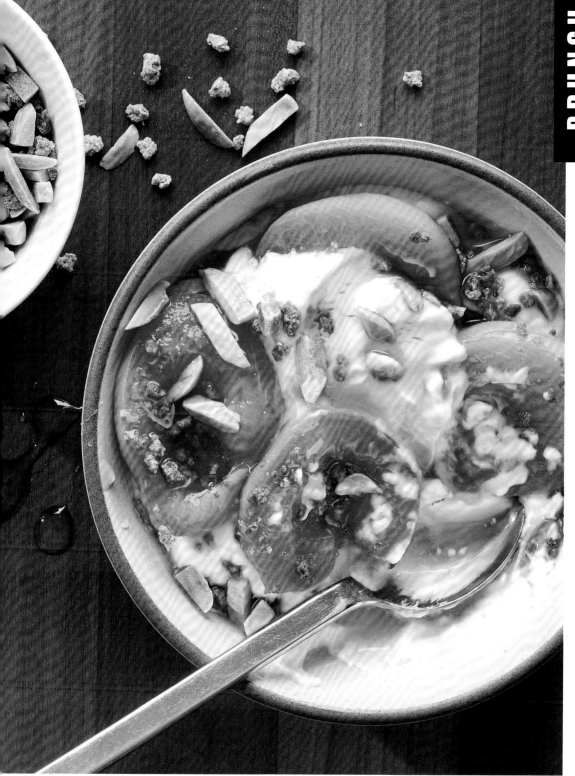

TUSCAN SAUSAGE AND KALE FRITTATA

TOTAL TIME: 40 MIN

WHAT YOU'LL NEED

12	large eggs
½	cup whole milk
2	oz pecorino cheese, grated (about ½ cup)
¼	tsp kosher salt
½	tsp pepper
2	Tbsp olive oil
1	small onion, finely chopped
½	lb Italian sausage, casings removed
½	large bunch kale, stems discarded and leaves chopped (about 3 cups)
1	cup marinara sauce
6	oz fresh mozzarella, sliced

Fresh basil leaves, for topping

HOW TO MAKE IT

■ Heat the oven to 350°F.

■ In a large bowl, whisk together the eggs, milk, pecorino, salt, and pepper.

■ In a large oven-safe skillet (preferably cast-iron) on medium, heat the oil. Add the onions and cook, covered, stirring occasionally, until tender, 5 minutes. Add the sausage and cook, breaking it up with a spoon, until browned, about 5 minutes. Add the kale and cook, stirring occasionally, until just wilted, about 1 minute.

■ Reduce heat to low and add the egg mixture, stirring to distribute the sausage and vegetables. Transfer the skillet to the oven and bake until almost set, 18 to 20 minutes. Remove from oven and heat the broiler.

■ Gently spread the sauce over the frittata then top with mozzarella. Broil until the cheese is browned and bubbling, 5 minutes. Top with basil and serve immediately.

MAKES 6 SERVINGS.

NUTRITION PER SERVING

480 calories

28 g protein

8 g carbohydrates (2 g fiber)

37 g fat

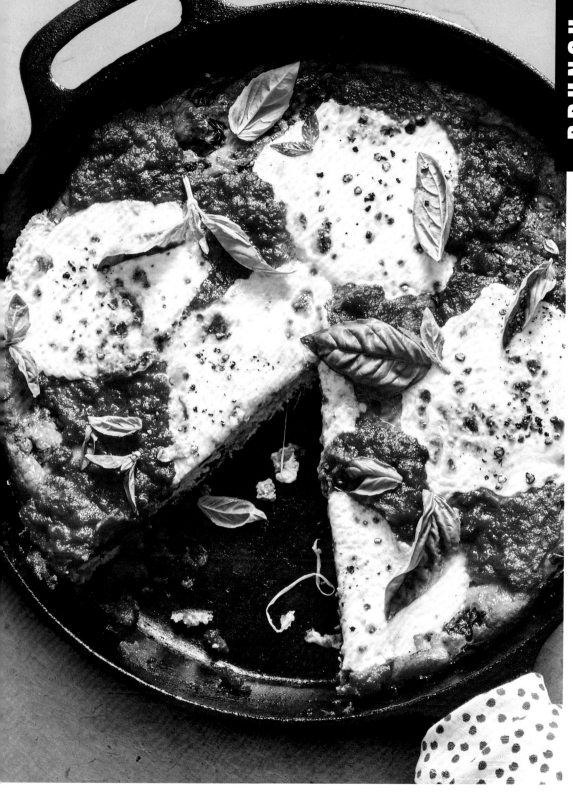

BAGEL BREAKFAST BAKE

TOTAL TIME: 1 HR 15 MIN

WHAT YOU'LL NEED

- 4 "everything" bagels, toasted and chopped
- 6 large eggs
- 2 cups milk
- 4 oz Monterey Jack cheese, shredded
- 4 slices cooked bacon, finely chopped
- 4 green onions, sliced, plus more for garnish
- ½ tsp salt
- ¼ tsp pepper

HOW TO MAKE IT

- ■ Arrange the bagel pieces in a 2- to 2½-qt baking dish.

- ■ In a large bowl, whisk together the eggs, milk, cheese, bacon, onions, salt and pepper. Pour the mixture over the bagels, pressing down slightly to submerge. Cover and refrigerate 1 hour or up to overnight.

- ■ Preheat the oven to 350°F. Uncover the dish and bake 45 to 55 minutes until set.

- ■ Let cool 15 minutes before serving; garnish with green onion.

MAKES 5 SERVINGS.

NUTRITION PER SERVING

466 calories

27 g protein

46 g carbohydrates (2 g fiber)

19 g fat

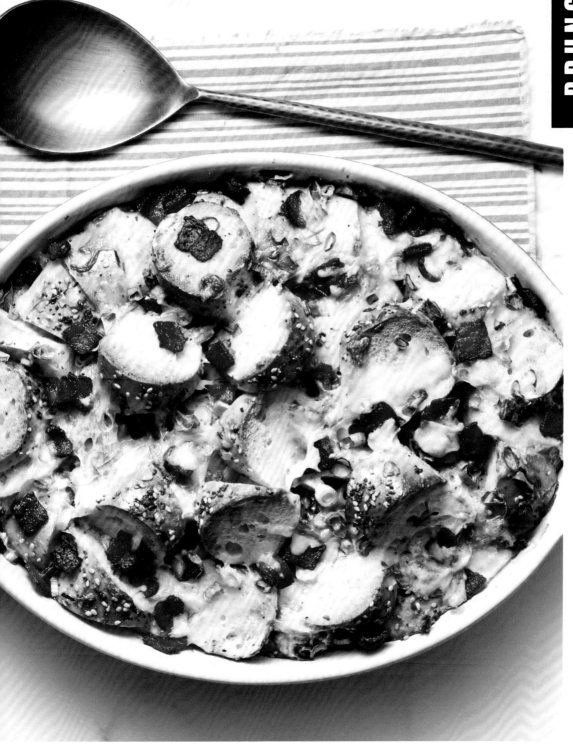

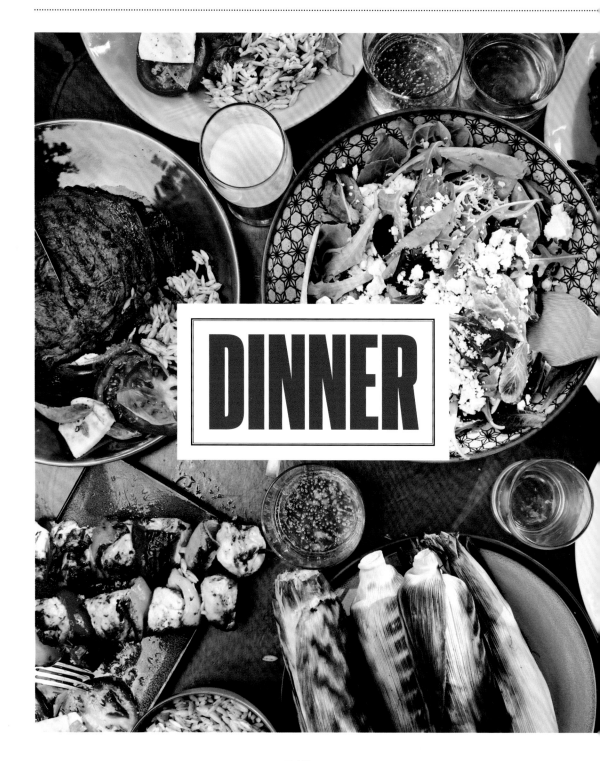

DINNER

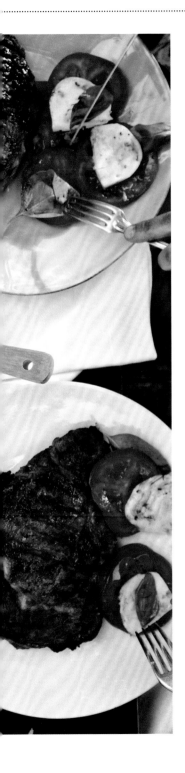

■ RECIPES

TURKEY TACOS

TOTAL TIME: 25 MIN

WHAT YOU'LL NEED

2	tsp oil
1	small red onion, chopped
1	clove garlic, finely chopped
1	lb extra-lean ground turkey
1	Tbsp sodium-free taco seasoning
8	whole-grain corn tortillas, warmed
¼	cup sour cream
½	cup shredded Mexican cheese
1	avocado, sliced
Salsa, for serving	
1	cup chopped lettuce

HOW TO MAKE IT

■ In a large skillet on medium high, heat the oil. Add the onion and cook, stirring until tender, 5 to 6 minutes. Stir in the garlic and cook 1 minute.

■ Add the turkey and cook, breaking it up with a spoon, until nearly brown, 5 minutes. Add the taco seasoning and 1 cup water. Simmer until reduced by slightly more than half, 7 minutes.

■ Fill the tortillas with turkey and top with sour cream, cheese, avocado, salsa, and lettuce.

MAKES 4 SERVINGS.

NUTRITION PER SERVING

472 calories

28 g protein

30 g carbohydrates (6 g fiber)

27 g fat

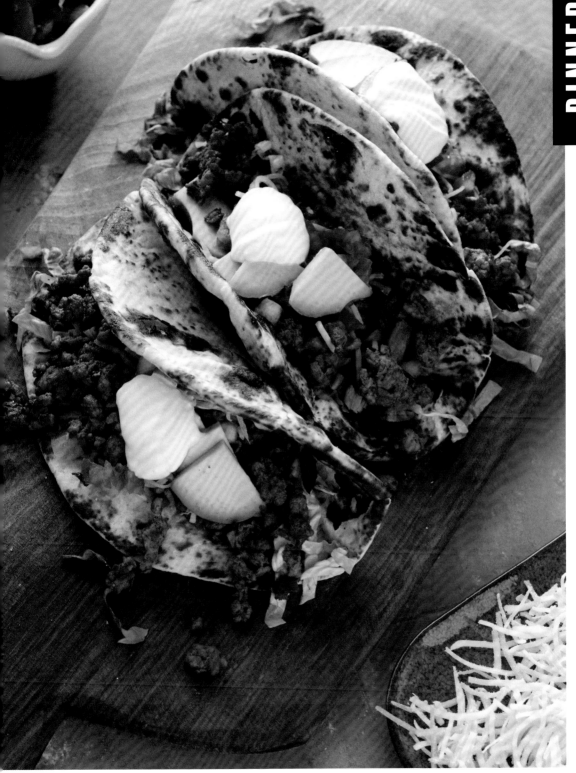

HEALTHY SPAGHETTI BOLOGNESE

TOTAL TIME: 1 HR 30 MIN

WHAT YOU'LL NEED

1   large spaghetti squash

3   Tbsp olive oil

½   tsp garlic powder

Kosher salt and pepper

1   small onion, finely chopped

1¼   lb ground turkey

4   cloves garlic, finely chopped

8   oz small cremini mushrooms, sliced

3   cups fresh diced tomatoes (or 2 15-oz cans)

1   (8-oz) can low-sodium, no-sugar-added tomato sauce

Fresh chopped basil

NUTRITION PER SERVING

450 calories

32 g protein

31 g carbohydrates (6 g fiber)

23 g fat

HOW TO MAKE IT

■ Preheat the oven to 400°F.

■ Cut the spaghetti squash in half lengthwise and discard seeds. Rub each half with ½ Tbsp oil and season with garlic powder and ¼ tsp each salt and pepper. Place skin-side up on a rimmed baking sheet and roast until tender, 35 to 40 minutes. Let cool for 10 minutes.

■ Meanwhile, in a large skillet on medium, heat remaining 2 Tbsp oil. Add the onion, season with ¼ tsp each salt and pepper, and cook, stirring occasionally, until tender, 6 minutes. Add the turkey and cook, breaking it up into small pieces with a spoon, until browned, 6 to 7 minutes. Stir in the garlic and cook 1 minute.

■ Push the turkey mixture to one side of the pan, and add the mushrooms to the other. Cook, stirring occasionally, until the mushrooms are tender, 5 minutes. Mix into the turkey.

■ Add the tomatoes and tomato sauce and simmer for 10 minutes.

■ While the sauce is simmering, scoop out the squash and transfer to plates. Spoon the turkey Bolognese over the top and sprinkle with basil, if desired.

MAKES 4 SERVINGS.

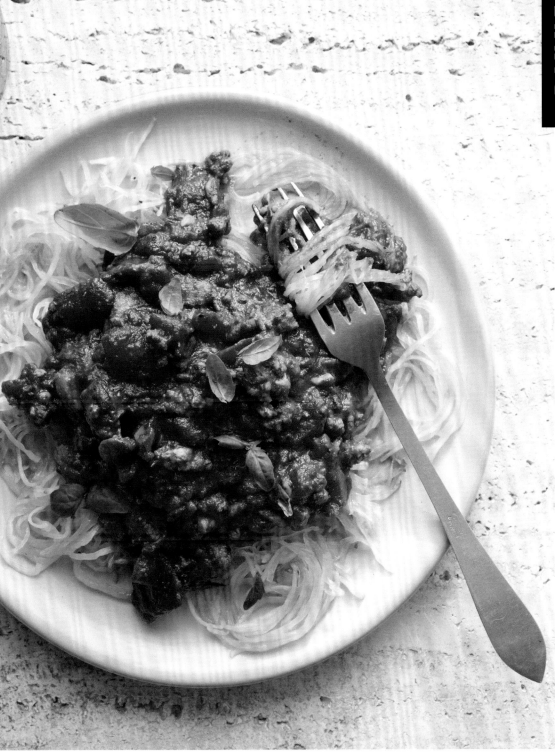

CHICKEN
with Fried Cauliflower Rice

TOTAL TIME: 35 MIN

WHAT YOU'LL NEED

- 2   Tbsp grapeseed oil
- 1¼   lb boneless, skinless chicken breast, pounded to even thickness
- 4   large eggs, beaten
- 2   red bell peppers, finely chopped
- 2   small carrots, finely chopped
- 1   onion, finely chopped
- 2   cloves garlic, finely chopped
- 4   scallions, finely chopped, plus more for serving
- ½   cup frozen peas, thawed
- 4   cups cauliflower "rice"
- 2   Tbsp low-sodium soy sauce
- 2   tsp rice vinegar

Kosher salt and pepper

NUTRITION PER SERVING

427 calories

45 g protein

25 g carbohydrates (7 g fiber)

16 g fat

HOW TO MAKE IT

- In a large, deep skillet over medium-high, heat 1 Tbsp oil. Add the chicken and cook until golden brown, 3 to 4 minutes per side. Transfer to a cutting board and let rest for 6 minutes before slicing.

- Add remaining 1 Tbsp oil to the skillet. Add the eggs and scramble until just set, 1 to 2 minutes; transfer to a bowl.

- To the skillet, add the bell pepper, carrot, and onion and cook, stirring often until just tender, 4 to 5 minutes. Stir in the garlic and cook, 1 minute. Toss with scallions and peas.

- Add the cauliflower, soy sauce, rice vinegar, salt and pepper and toss to combine. Then let the cauliflower sit, without stirring, until beginning to brown, 2 to 3 minutes. Toss with the sliced chicken and eggs.

MAKES 4 SERVINGS.

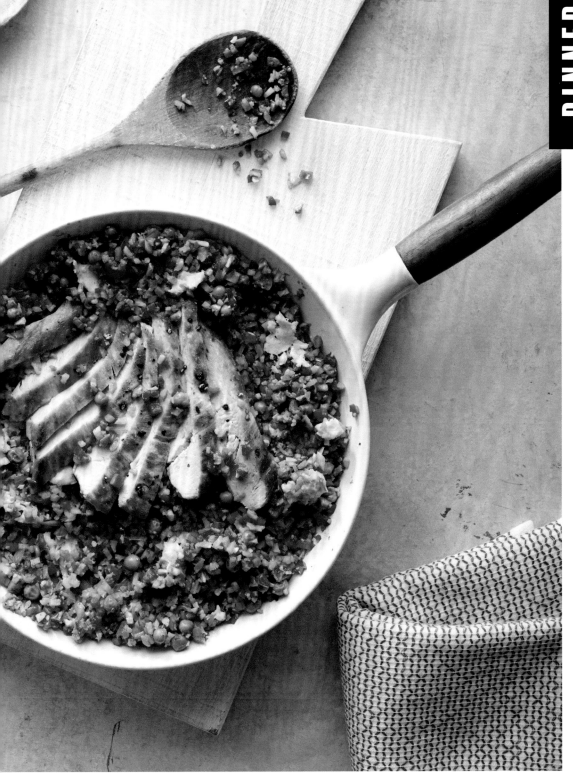

SHEET PAN STEAK
with Beans and Broccolini

TOTAL TIME: 50 MIN

WHAT YOU'LL NEED

1   lb small cremini mushrooms, trimmed and halved

1¼ lb bunch broccolini, trimmed and cut into 2-in. lengths

4   cloves garlic, finely chopped

3   Tbsp olive oil

¼   tsp red pepper flakes (or a bit more for extra kick)

Kosher salt and pepper

2   1-in.-thick New York strip steaks (about 1½ lb total), trimmed of excess fat

1   15-oz can low-sodium cannellini beans, rinsed

HOW TO MAKE IT

■ Preheat the oven to 450°F. On a large rimmed baking sheet, toss the mushrooms, broccolini, garlic, oil, red pepper flakes, and ¼ tsp each salt and pepper. Place the baking sheet in the oven and roast 15 minutes.

■ Push the mixture to the edges of the pan to make room for the steaks. Season the steaks with ¼ tsp each salt and pepper and place in the center of the pan. Roast the steaks to desired doneness, 5 to 7 minutes per side for medium-rare. Transfer the steaks to a cutting board and let rest 5 minutes before slicing.

■ Add the beans to the baking sheet and toss to combine. Roast until heated through, about 3 minutes. Serve beans and vegetables with steak.

MAKES 4 SERVINGS.

NUTRITION PER SERVING

464 calories

42 g protein

26 g carbohydrates (8 g fiber)

22 g fat

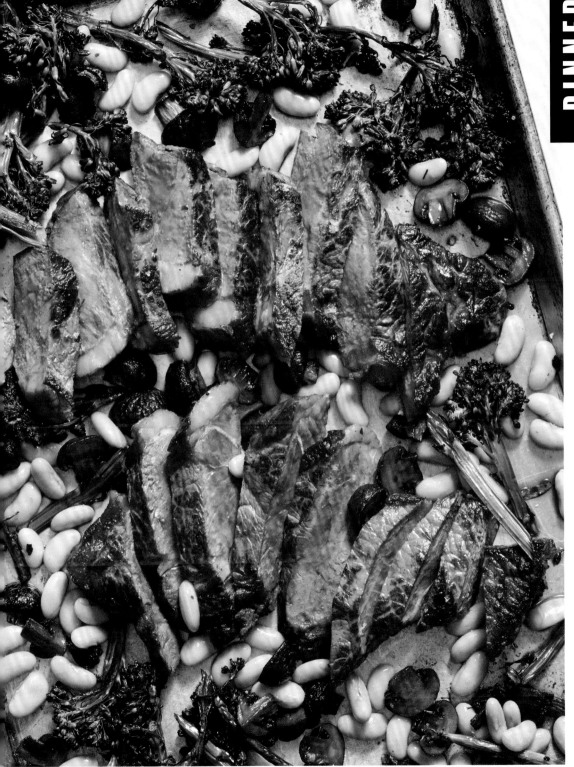

PORK TENDERLOIN
with Butternut Squash and Brussels Sprouts

TOTAL TIME: 50 MIN

WHAT YOU'LL NEED

1¾ lb pork tenderloin, trimmed

Salt

Pepper

3   Tbsp canola oil

2   sprigs fresh thyme

2   garlic cloves, peeled

4   cups Brussels sprouts, trimmed and halved

4   cups diced butternut squash

HOW TO MAKE IT

■ Preheat the oven to 400°F. Season the tenderloin all over with salt and pepper. In a large cast-iron pan over medium high, heat 1 Tbsp oil. When the oil shimmers, add the tenderloin and sear until golden brown on all sides, 8 to 12 minutes total. Transfer to a plate.

■ Add the thyme and garlic and remaining 2 Tbsp oil to the pan and cook until aromatic, about 1 minute. Add the Brussels sprouts, the butternut squash, and a big pinch each of salt and pepper. Cook, stirring occasionally, until the vegetables are slightly browned, 4 to 6 minutes. Place the tenderloin atop the vegetables and transfer everything to the oven.

■ Roast until the vegetables are tender and a meat thermometer inserted into the thickest part of the tenderloin registers 140°F, 15 to 20 minutes.

■ Wearing oven mitts, carefully remove the pan from the oven. Allow the tenderloin to rest 5 minutes before slicing and serving with the vegetables. Toss greens with a balsamic vinaigrette to serve as a side.

MAKES 4 SERVINGS.

NUTRITION PER SERVING

401 calories

44 g protein

25 g carbohydrates
(6 g fiber)

15 g fat

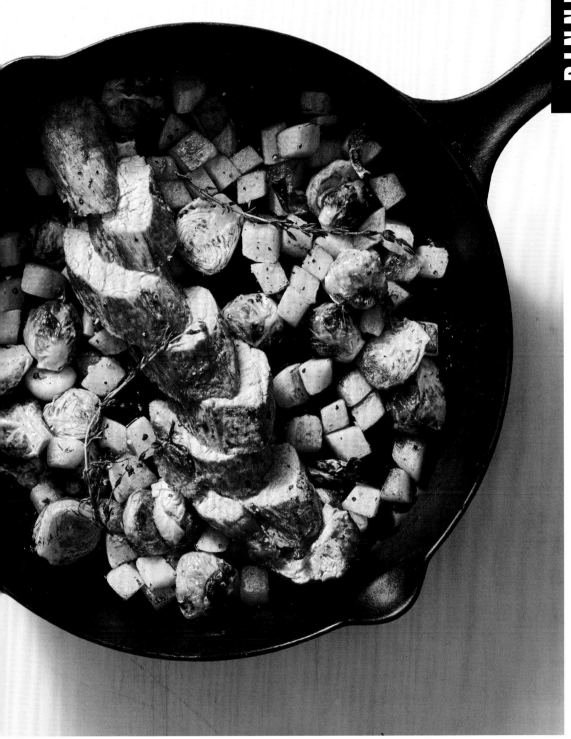

WILD CAJUN SPICED SALMON

TOTAL TIME: 30 MIN

WHAT YOU'LL NEED

1½ lb wild Alaskan salmon fillet

Sodium-free taco seasoning

½ head cauliflower (about 1 lb), cut into florets

1 head broccoli (about 1 lb), cut into florets

3 Tbsp olive oil

½ tsp garlic powder

4 medium tomatoes, diced

HOW TO MAKE IT

■ Preheat the oven to 375°F. Place the salmon in a baking dish.

■ In a small bowl, mix the taco seasoning with ½ cup water. Pour the mixture over the salmon and bake until opaque throughout, 12 to 15 minutes.

■ Meanwhile, in a food processor (in batches as necessary), pulse the cauliflower and broccoli until finely chopped and "riced."

■ In a large skillet on medium, heat the oil. Add the cauliflower and broccoli, sprinkle with garlic powder, and cook, tossing until just tender, 5 to 6 minutes.

■ Serve salmon on top of "rice" and top with tomatoes.

MAKES 4 SERVINGS.

NUTRITION PER SERVING

408 calories

42 g protein

9 g carbohydrates (3 g fiber)

23 g fat

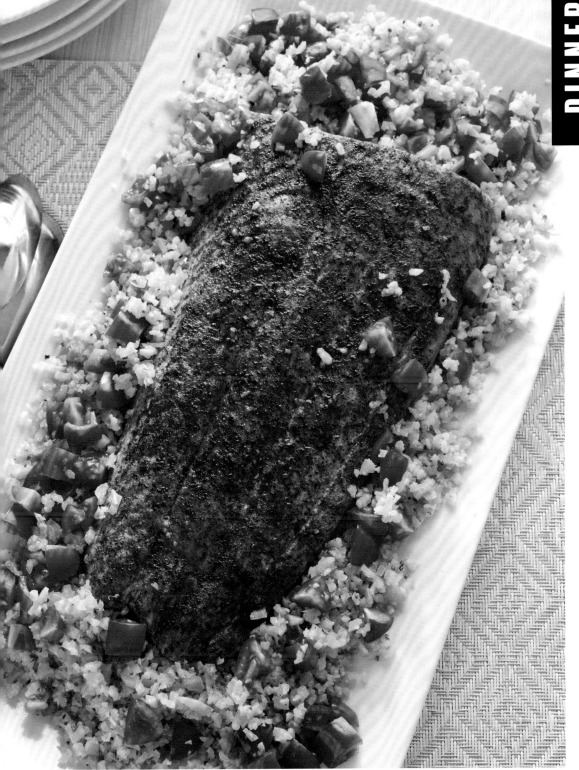

PORK CHOPS
with Bloody Mary Tomato Salad

TOTAL TIME: 25 MIN

WHAT YOU'LL NEED

- 2 Tbsp olive oil
- 2 Tbsp red wine vinegar
- 2 tsp Worcestershire sauce
- 2 tsp prepared horseradish, squeezed dry
- ½ tsp Tabasco
- ½ tsp celery seeds

Kosher salt

- 1 pint cherry tomatoes, halved
- 2 celery stalks, very thinly sliced
- ½ small red onion, thinly sliced
- 4 small bone-in pork chops (1 in. thick, about 2¼ lb total)

Pepper

- ¼ cup finely chopped flat-leaf parsley
- 1 small head green-leaf lettuce, leaves torn

NUTRITION PER SERVING

400 calories

39 g protein

8 g carbohydrates (3 g fiber)

23 g fat

HOW TO MAKE IT

■ Heat grill to medium high. In a large bowl, whisk together the oil, vinegar, Worcestershire sauce, horseradish, Tabasco, celery seeds, and ¼ tsp salt. Toss with the tomatoes, celery, and onion.

■ Season the pork chops with ½ tsp each salt and pepper and grill until golden brown and just cooked through, 5 to 7 minutes per side.

■ Fold the parsley into the tomatoes and serve over pork and greens. Eat with mashed cauliflower or potatoes.

MAKES 4 SERVINGS.

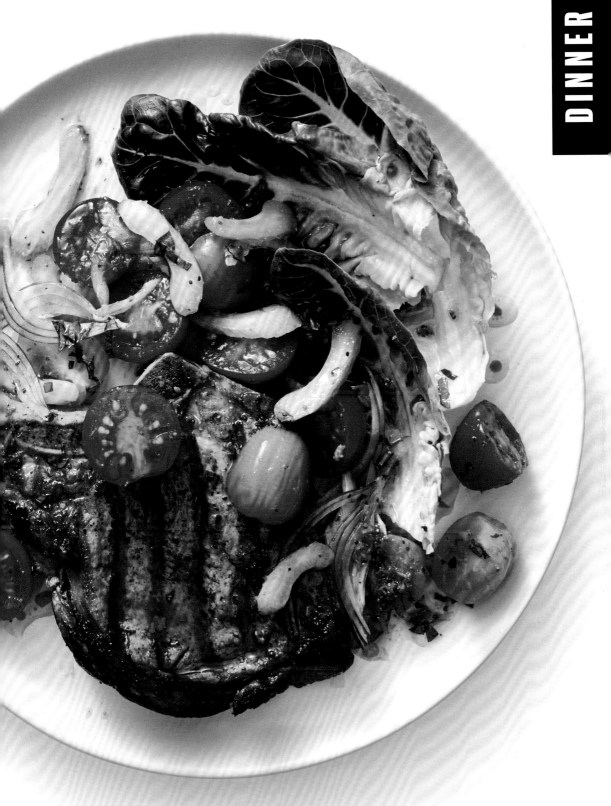

ROASTED COD AND NEW POTATOES
with Chorizo Vinaigrette

TOTAL TIME: 30 MIN

WHAT YOU'LL NEED

4   Tbsp plus 1 tsp olive oil

2   lb yellow new potatoes, halved

Salt

Pepper

4   6-oz pieces cod fillet

2   oz chorizo, finely chopped

1   shallot, finely chopped

2   Tbsp sherry vinegar

Parsley, for garnish

HOW TO MAKE IT

■ Preheat the oven to 450°F. Coat a rimmed baking sheet with 3 Tbsp olive oil. Season the potatoes with salt and pepper and place them cut-sides down on the baking sheet. Roast for 15 minutes.

■ Pat the cod fillets dry with paper towel and season with ¼ tsp each salt and pepper. Place the cod on the sheet pan with the potatoes, moving the potatoes aside as necessary. Roast until the cod is opaque throughout, 7 to 9 minutes.

■ Meanwhile, in a small skillet on medium, heat 1 Tbsp olive oil. Add the chorizo and cook until crispy, 2 to 3 minutes.

■ Remove the skillet from heat and add the shallot.

■ Stir in the sherry vinegar. Serve over fish and potatoes and sprinkle with parsley.

MAKES 4 SERVINGS.

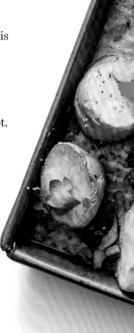

NUTRITION PER SERVING

472 calories

35 g protein

37 g carbohydrates (4 g fiber)

20 g fat

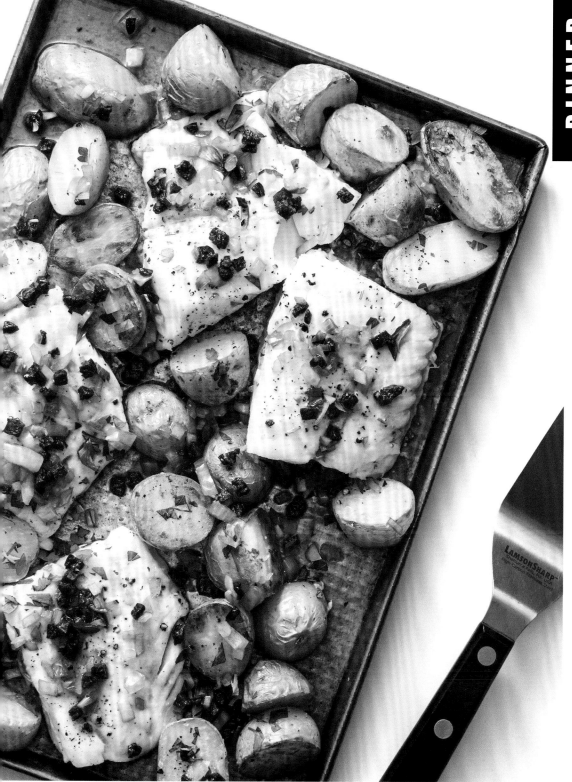

GRILLED CHICKEN
with Smoky Corn Salad

TOTAL TIME: 30 MIN

WHAT YOU'LL NEED

4   6-oz boneless, skinless chicken breast halves

Salt

Pepper

2   limes, halved

5   ears corn, shucked

¼   cup chopped cilantro

2   Tbsp chopped green olives

2   oz Manchego cheese, finely grated

2½ tsp olive oil

1   tsp smoked paprika

HOW TO MAKE IT

■ Season the boneless, skinless chicken breast halves with salt and pepper and grill on medium high to cook through, 5 to 6 minutes per side.

■ Meanwhile, grill the limes, cut-sides down, and corn until charred, 6 to 8 minutes.

■ Cut the corn from the cob and toss into a medium bowl with juice of 2 lime halves, cilantro, olives, cheese, and pinch each salt and pepper.

■ Serve the chicken with the corn and remaining lime halves, and drizzle with a mixture of olive oil and smoked paprika. Eat with half an avocado for an extra dose of hunger-crushing healthy fats.

MAKES 4 SERVINGS.

NUTRITION PER SERVING

458 calories

46 g protein

25 g carbohydrates (3 g fiber)

20 g fat

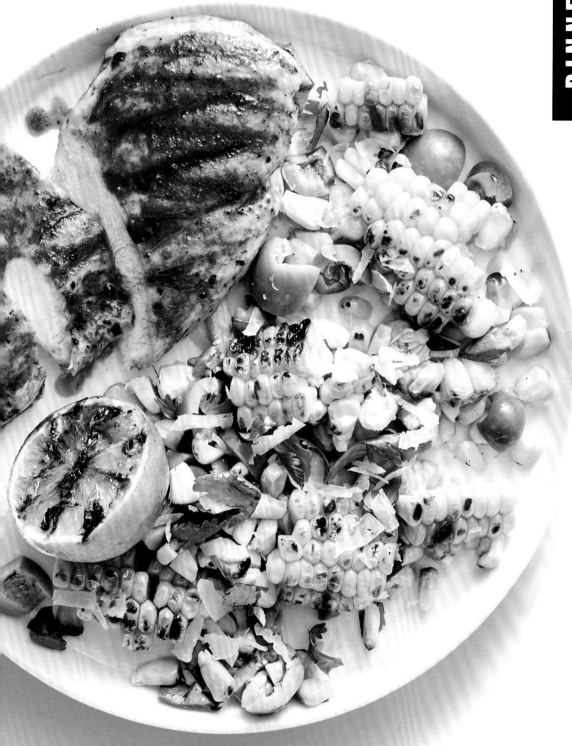

GRILLED AHI TUNA
over Mashed Cauliflower

TOTAL TIME: 20 MIN

WHAT YOU'LL NEED

1	medium head cauliflower, cut into small florets (about 7 cups)
4	Tbsp extra-virgin olive oil
2	Tbsp fresh lemon juice
1	Tbsp capers, roughly chopped
10	cups baby power green mix
24	oz sashimi tuna (sushi grade), cut into 4 portions
½	tsp fine sea salt
¼	tsp ground black pepper

HOW TO MAKE IT

■ Fill a large pot with 2 in. water, place a steamer basket on top, and bring water to a boil. Add the cauliflower, cover, and steam until very tender, 8 to 10 minutes. Transfer the cauliflower to a food processor and the steaming water to a measuring cup. Add 2 Tbsp oil and puree, adding reserved cooking liquid 1 Tbsp at a time until smooth.

■ While the cauliflower is steaming, heat the grill or grill pan on medium high.

■ In a small bowl, combine the lemon juice, remaining 2 Tbsp oil, capers, and pinch each salt and pepper. Arrange greens on a platter.

■ Lightly oil the grill. Season the tuna with ½ tsp salt and ½ tsp pepper, grill until charred, 1½ minutes per side. Transfer to a cutting board and let rest at least 3 minutes before slicing.

■ Spoon the cauliflower on top of the greens and the sliced tuna on top of that, then spoon the vinaigrette over the top.

MAKES 4 SERVINGS.

NUTRITION PER SERVING

434 calories

46 g protein

12 g carbohydrates (6 g fiber)

23 g fat

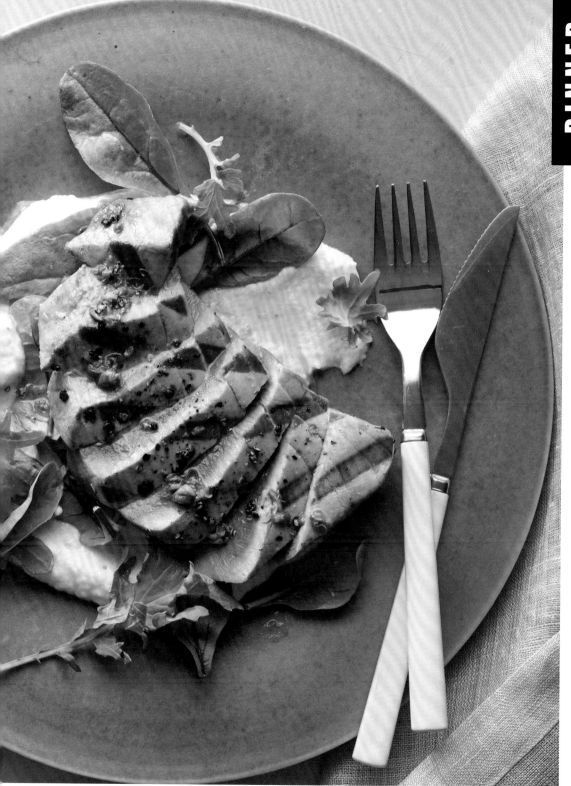

ASIAN TOFU
with Baby Bok Choy

TOTAL TIME: 1 HR

WHAT YOU'LL NEED

2 14-oz package extra-firm tofu

3 Tbsp low-sodium soy sauce

2 Tbsp chili garlic sauce

2 cloves garlic, pressed

2 tsp honey

3 Tbsp toasted sesame oil

Vegetable oil, for baking sheet

8 small heads baby bok choy, trimmed and halved

4 cups sugar snap peas, thinly sliced

1 tsp black sesame seeds

HOW TO MAKE IT

■ Place the tofu on a rimmed baking sheet between paper towels. Top with another baking sheet and weigh down with heavy cans or skillet; let sit 30 minutes.

■ Meanwhile, combine the soy sauce, chili garlic sauce, garlic, honey, and 2 Tbsp sesame oil.

■ Preheat the oven to 400°F. Transfer the tofu to a cutting board. Wipe off the baking sheet and lightly coat with vegetable oil. Slice the tofu into ½-in.-thick triangles and arrange on prepared sheet. Drizzle with 2 Tbsp sauce mixture and bake until top is golden, 12 to 15 minutes.

■ Turn the tofu over, arrange on one side of the baking sheet, and drizzle with 2 Tbsp sauce mixture. Arrange the bok choy on the other half of the sheet and gently toss with remaining 1 Tbsp sesame oil.

■ Roast until the tofu is golden brown and bok choy is tender, 8 to 12 minutes. Drizzle remaining sauce over the tofu and sprinkle everything with snap peas and sesame seeds. Serve over brown rice.

MAKES 4 SERVINGS.

NUTRITION PER SERVING

369 calories

25 g protein

21 g carbohydrates (7 g fiber)

21 g fat

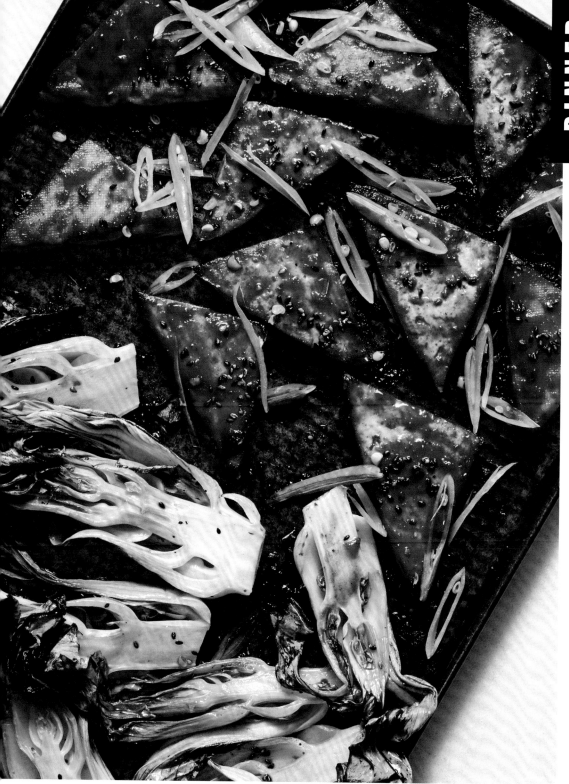

WHITE BEAN AND TUNA SALAD
with Basil Vinaigrette

TOTAL TIME: 25 MIN

WHAT YOU'LL NEED

Kosher salt and pepper

12	oz green beans, trimmed and halved
1	small shallot, chopped
1	cup lightly packed basil leaves
3	Tbsp olive oil
1	Tbsp red wine vinegar
4	cups torn lettuce
1	15-oz can small white beans, rinsed
2	5-oz cans solid white tuna in water, drained
3	soft-boiled eggs, halved

HOW TO MAKE IT

■ Bring a large pot of water to a boil. Add 1 Tbsp salt and then the green beans, and cook until just tender, 3 to 4 minutes. Drain and rinse under cold water to cool.

■ Meanwhile, in a blender, puree the shallot, basil, oil, vinegar, and ½ tsp each salt and pepper until smooth.

■ Transfer half of the dressing to a large bowl and toss with the green beans. Fold in the lettuce, white beans, and tuna and serve with remaining dressing and eggs.

MAKES 3 SERVINGS.

NUTRITION PER SERVING

463 calories

35 g protein

34 g carbohydrates (10 g fiber)

22 g fat

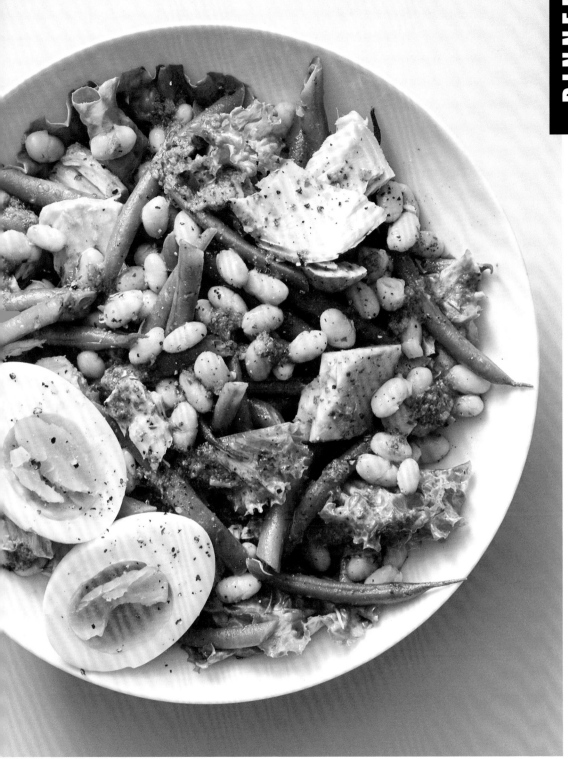

SPEEDY FISH TACOS

TOTAL TIME: 23 MIN

WHAT YOU'LL NEED

1   large white onion, thinly sliced

1   jalapeño pepper, finely chopped

2   Tbsp lime juice

2   Tbsp chopped fresh cilantro

½   tsp salt

2½   Tbsp canola oil

1½   lb halibut fillet

1   tsp chili powder

1   tsp ground cumin

12   corn tortillas

2   cups shredded romaine lettuce

1   medium tomato, chopped

1   avocado, sliced

HOW TO MAKE IT

■ In a medium bowl, combine the onion, jalapeño, lime juice, cilantro, 1 Tbsp oil and ¼ tsp salt.

■ In a large nonstick skillet over medium high, heat remaining 1½ Tbsp oil. Sprinkle the halibut with the chili powder, cumin, and remaining ¼ tsp salt. Add the fish to the skillet and cook until the fish flakes easily with a fork, about 5 to 6 minutes per side. Remove from the skillet.

■ Heat the tortillas according to package directions. Fill the tortillas with the halibut, lettuce, tomato, and avocado. Top with the onion mixture.

MAKES 4 SERVINGS.

NUTRITION PER SERVING

510 calories

37 g protein

44 g carbohydrate (8 g fiber)

21 g fat

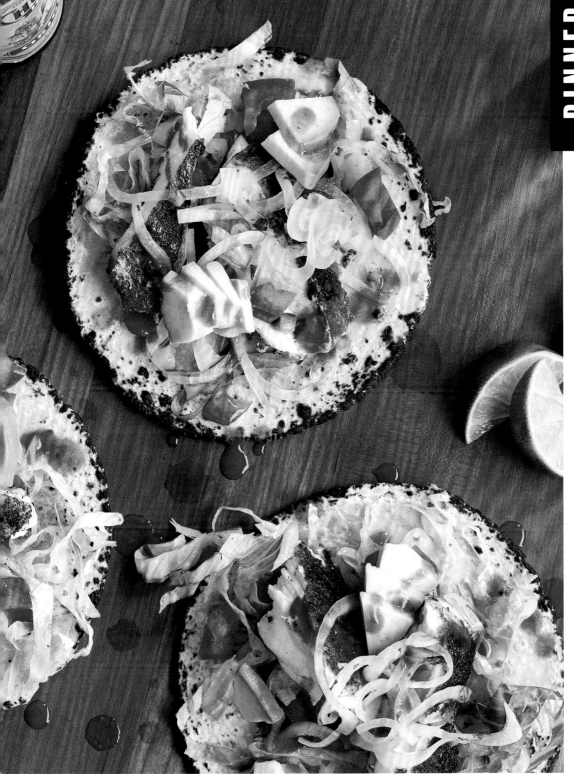

TUNA AND CHEDDAR WRAPS

TOTAL TIME: 10 MIN

WHAT YOU'LL NEED

4	(3-oz) tuna fish pouches
¼	cup olive oil mayonnaise
2	scallions, chopped
1	red bell pepper, finely chopped
2	tsp olive oil
4	medium whole-grain tortillas
4	oz sharp Cheddar, coarsely grated
8	pieces butter lettuce
2	cups grape tomatoes, sliced

HOW TO MAKE IT

■ In a large bowl, combine the tuna, mayo, scallions, and bell pepper.

■ In a large nonstick skillet on medium, heat 1 tsp oil. Working with 2 tortillas at a time, cook until beginning to brown, flip, and top with half the cheese; cook until melted. Transfer to plates and repeat with remaining 1 tsp oil, tortillas, and cheese.

■ Divide the tuna mixture among the tortillas, and then top with lettuce and tomatoes and wrap up. Eat with hummus and baby carrots, fruit and yogurt, or a small bowl of soup.

MAKES 4 SERVINGS.

NUTRITION PER SERVING

360 calories

29 g protein

22 g carbohydrates (5 g fiber)

17 g fat

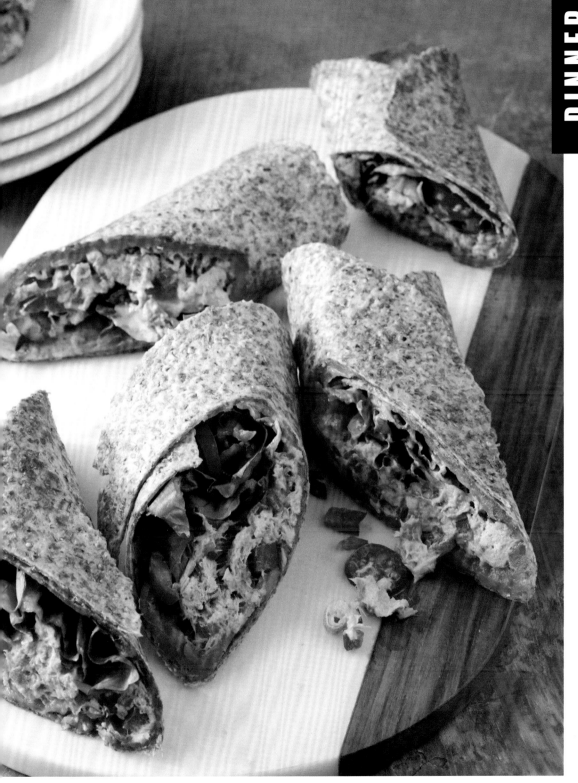

ROASTED SWEET POTATO AND CHICKEN SALAD

TOTAL TIME: 30 MIN

WHAT YOU'LL NEED

2½ lb sweet potatoes, cut into ½-in. chunks

2 Tbsp olive oil

¼ tsp salt

¼ cup seasoned rice vinegar

2 Tbsp toasted sesame oil

1 Tbsp miso paste

1 Tbsp finely chopped peeled fresh ginger

¼ tsp pepper

20 oz mixed greens

2 rotisserie chicken breast halves (about 8 oz), sliced

1 avocado, sliced

Sesame seeds, for garnish

NUTRITION PER SERVING

480 calories

21 g protein

48 g carbohydrates (11 g fiber)

24 g fat

HOW TO MAKE IT

■ Preheat the oven to 450°F. On a large rimmed baking sheet, toss the sweet potatoes with olive oil and salt. Roast for 25 minutes or until tender.

■ In a small bowl, whisk together the rice vinegar, sesame oil, miso, ginger, and pepper.

■ Among four plates layered with 5 oz mixed greens, divide the sweet potatoes, rotisserie chicken, and avocado. Drizzle with miso vinaigrette; top with sesame seeds.

MAKES 4 SERVINGS.

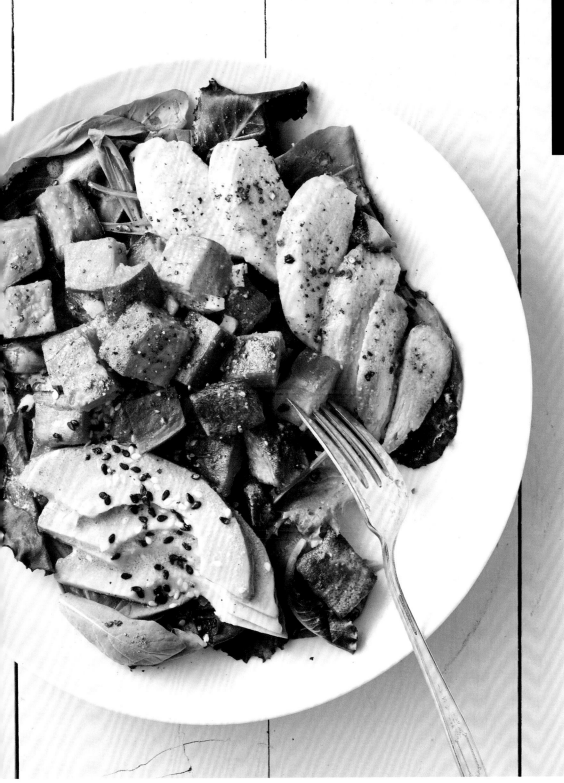

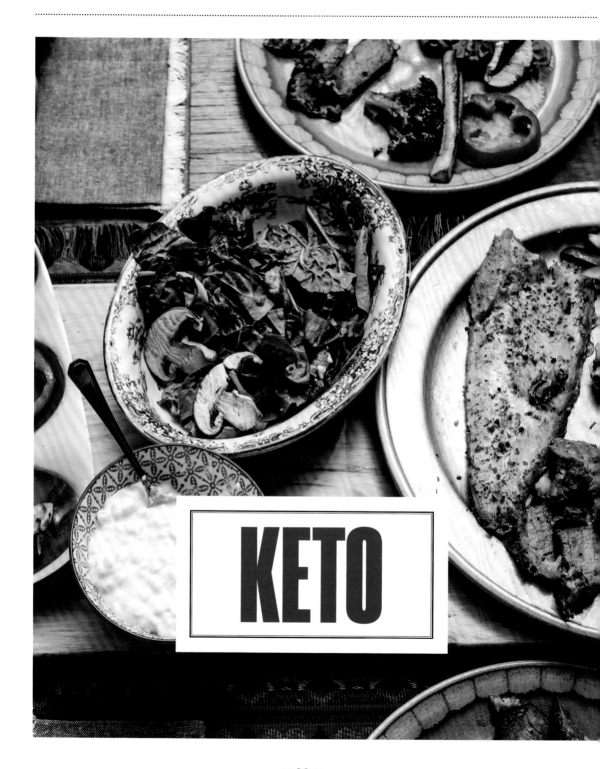

KETO

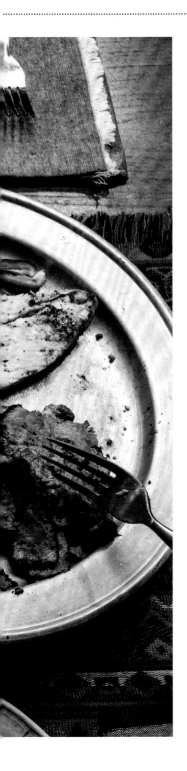

■ RECIPES

BACON WRAPPED MEATLOAF

TOTAL TIME: 1 HR 15 MIN

WHAT YOU'LL NEED

Cooking spray

1	Tbsp extra-virgin olive oil
1	medium onion, chopped
1	stalk celery, chopped
3	cloves garlic, minced
1	tsp dried oregano
1	tsp chili powder
2	lbs ground beef
1	cup shredded Cheddar
½	cup almond flour
¼	cup grated Parmesan
2	eggs
1	Tbsp low-sodium soy sauce

Kosher salt

Freshly ground black pepper

6	thin strips bacon

NUTRITION PER SERVING

450 calories

46 g protein

6 g carbohydrates
(2 g fiber)

27 g fat

HOW TO MAKE IT

■ Preheat oven to 400°F. Grease a medium baking dish with cooking spray. In a medium skillet over medium, heat oil. Add onion and celery and cook until soft, 5 minutes. Stir in garlic, oregano, and chili powder and cook until fragrant, 1 minute. Let mixture cool slightly.

■ In a large bowl, combine ground beef, vegetable mixture, cheese, almond flour, Parmesan, eggs, soy sauce, and season with salt and pepper. Shape into a large loaf in baking dish, then lay bacon slices on top.

■ Cook until bacon is crispy and beef is cooked through, about 1 hour. If bacon is cooking too quickly, cover dish with foil.

MAKES 6 SERVINGS.

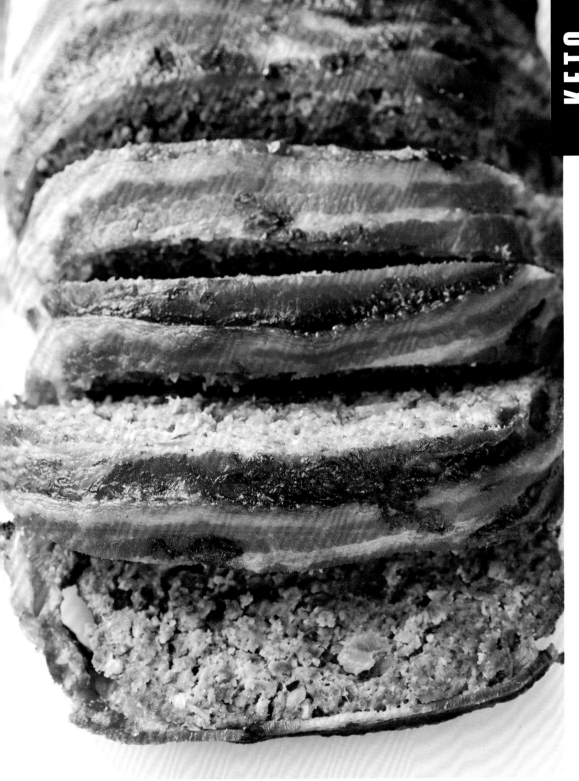

BUNLESS BACON, EGG & CHEESE

TOTAL TIME: 10 MIN

WHAT YOU'LL NEED

Cooking spray

2 eggs

2 Tbsp water

½ avocado, lightly mashed

2 slices cooked bacon

¼ cup shredded Cheddar cheese

HOW TO MAKE IT

■ In a medium nonstick pan, place two mason jar lids (centers removed). Spray the entire pan with cooking spray and heat over medium. Crack eggs into the centers of the lids and lightly whisk with a fork to break up yolk.

■ Pour water around the lids and cover the pan. Cook, letting the eggs steam, until the whites are cooked through, about 3 minutes. Remove lid and top one of the eggs with Cheddar. Cook until the cheese is slightly melty, about 1 minute more.

■ Invert the egg bun without the cheese onto the plate. Top with mashed avocado, cooked bacon, and the cheesy egg bun, cheese side-down. Eat with fork and knife.

MAKES 1 SERVING.

NUTRITION PER SERVING

460 calories

27 g protein

7 g carbohydrates (5 g fiber)

36 g fat

CHILEAN SEA BASS
with Spinach-Avocado Pesto

TOTAL TIME: 30 MIN

WHAT YOU'LL NEED

4 wild Chilean sea bass fillets, about 2 lbs

Kosher salt

Freshly ground black pepper

2 cups baby spinach

½ cup fresh parsley, chopped, plus more for garnish

1 clove garlic, smashed

¼ cup walnuts, chopped

2 tsp fresh lemon juice

Extra-virgin olive oil

1 avocado, pitted

1 lb asparagus, ends trimmed

2 lemons, cut in half

Flaky sea salt

HOW TO MAKE IT

■ Season sea bass with kosher salt and pepper; set aside.

■ In the bowl of a food processor, add spinach, parsley, garlic, walnuts, lemon juice, ¼ cup olive oil, ½ tsp kosher salt and ¼ tsp pepper. Pulse 2 to 3 times. Add avocado and pulse until the sauce is well blended but still maintaining some texture.

■ Preheat a large cast-iron skillet over high. Heat 1 Tbsp olive oil until very hot and almost smoking. Sear sea bass on each side for 3 minutes. Transfer to a plate and let rest for 1 minute.

■ Meanwhile, return cast-iron skillet to medium-high. Add 1 tsp olive oil, asparagus, and ½ tsp kosher salt. Sauté for 5 minutes, then transfer asparagus to a plate for serving. Place lemons cut-side down in the skillet, turn heat to high, and sear for 1 minute.

■ Serve sea bass on bed of asparagus and top with pesto and seared lemon.

■ Garnish with parsley and sprinkle of sea salt.

MAKES 4 SERVINGS.

NUTRITION PER SERVING

410 calories

58 g protein

10 g carbohydrates (6 g fiber)

15 g fat

EGG ROLL BOWLS

TOTAL TIME: 35 MIN

WHAT YOU'LL NEED

- 1 Tbsp vegetable oil
- 1 clove garlic, minced
- 1 Tbsp minced fresh ginger
- 1 lb ground pork
- 1 Tbsp sesame oil
- ½ onion, thinly sliced
- 1 cup shredded carrot
- ¼ green cabbage, thinly sliced
- ¼ cup soy sauce
- 1 Tbsp Sriracha
- 1 green onion, thinly sliced
- 1 Tbsp sesame seeds

HOW TO MAKE IT

- In a large skillet over medium heat, heat vegetable oil. Add garlic and ginger and cook until fragrant, 1 to 2 minutes. Add pork and cook until no pink remains.

- Push pork to the side and add sesame oil. Add onion, carrot, and cabbage. Stir to combine with meat and add soy sauce and Sriracha. Cook until cabbage is tender, 5 to 8 minutes.

- Transfer mixture to a serving dish and garnish with green onions and sesame seeds.

MAKES 4 SERVINGS.

NUTRITION PER SERVING

420 calories

22 g protein

11 g carbohydrates (3 g fiber)

32 g fat

SPINACH-ARTICHOKE STUFFED MUSHROOMS

TOTAL TIME: 40 MIN

WHAT YOU'LL NEED

4   medium portobello mushrooms, stems and gills removed

2   Tbsp extra virgin olive oil

1   package frozen chopped spinach, thawed, drained and squeezed dry

1   (14-oz) can artichoke hearts, drained and chopped

¼   (8-oz) block cream cheese, cut into 20 pieces, room temperature

2   Tbsp mayonnaise

2   Tbsp sour cream

1   cup shredded mozzarella, divided

½   cup grated Parmesan, divided

2   cloves garlic, minced

Red pepper flakes

Kosher salt

Freshly ground black pepper

HOW TO MAKE IT

■ Preheat oven to 375°F. Brush face-down mushroom caps with olive oil. Cook on baking sheet for about 10 minutes until beginning to soften.

■ Meanwhile, combine spinach, artichoke, cream cheese, mayonnaise, sour cream, ½ cup mozzarella, ¼ cup Parmesan, garlic, and red pepper flakes in a large bowl. Season with salt and pepper to taste.

■ Flip over mushrooms and stuff each cap with an equal amount of the spinach mixture. Sprinkle tops with remaining cheeses.

■ Return pan to oven and bake for another 10 to 15 minutes, until the mushrooms are easily pierced with fork and the cheese is melted.

■ Once melted, switch oven to broil and broil the mushroom caps for a few minutes until the cheese starts to brown.

MAKES 4 SERVINGS.

NUTRITION PER SERVING

470 calories

17 g protein

16 g carbohydrates (5 g fiber)

39 g fat

CHEESY LASAGNA

TOTAL TIME: 1 HR

WHAT YOU'LL NEED

FOR THE "NOODLE" LAYER

- 3 large eggs
- 1 (12-oz) container riced cauliflower (about 2½ cups)
- 1 cup shredded mozzarella

Kosher salt

FOR THE MEAT FILLING

- ½ Tbsp extra-virgin olive oil
- 1 lb ground turkey
- 1 tsp Italian seasoning

Kosher salt

Freshly ground black pepper

- 2 Tbsp tomato paste
- ¾ cup crushed tomatoes

FOR THE CHEESE FILLING

- 1 cup ricotta cheese
- ¾ cup shredded mozzarella, divided
- ¼ cup grated Parmesan
- 1 large egg, beaten
- 1 tsp Italian seasoning

Kosher salt

Freshly ground black pepper

Freshly chopped parsley, for garnish

NUTRITION PER SERVING

500 calories

58 g protein

14 g carbohydrates (4 g fiber)

26 g fat

HOW TO MAKE IT

■ Preheat the oven to 350°F and line a rimmed half sheet pan with parchment paper. In a large bowl, beat eggs, then stir in cauliflower, 1 cup mozzarella, and salt. Spread cauliflower mixture onto prepared sheet pan in an even layer about ¾-in. thick.

■ Bake until firm to the touch and golden, 25 minutes. Let cool 10 minutes, and increase oven temperature to 400°F.

■ Meanwhile, in a medium skillet over medium-high heat, heat oil. Add ground turkey and season with Italian seasoning, salt, and pepper. Cook turkey, breaking up the meat with back of a wooden spoon, until no longer pink, 6 to 8 minutes. Stir in tomato paste and crushed tomatoes and cook 2 minutes, stirring constantly. Remove from heat.

■ In a medium bowl, mix ricotta cheese, ½ cup mozzarella, Parmesan, egg, and Italian seasoning until combined. Season with salt and pepper.

■ Grease an 8-in. square baking dish with cooking spray. Add half the meat to the baking pan. Cut the cauliflower "noodle" layer into strips and place in baking dish to fit bottom layer. Top with entire ricotta mixture and more cauliflower noodles, then top with remaining meat and cauliflower noodles. Sprinkle remaining ¼ cup shredded mozzarella on top. Bake in oven until golden, 20 to 25 minutes.

■ Garnish with parsley before serving.

MAKES 4 SERVINGS.

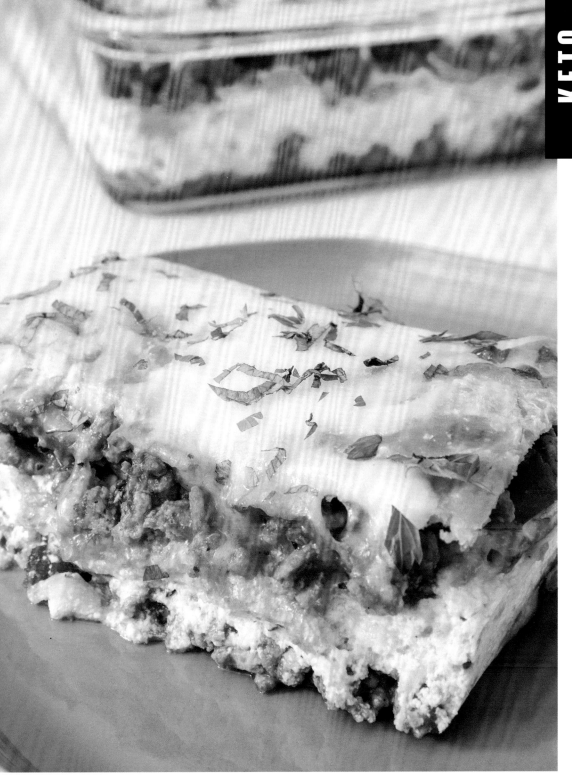

ROSEMARY-DIJON SALMON

TOTAL TIME: 20 MIN

WHAT YOU'LL NEED

1   Tbsp grainy mustard

2   cloves garlic, finely minced

1   Tbsp finely minced shallots

2   tsp fresh thyme leaves, chopped, plus more for garnish

2   tsp fresh rosemary, chopped

Juice of ½ lemon

Kosher salt

Freshly ground black pepper

4   (4-oz) salmon fillets

Lemon slices, for serving

HOW TO MAKE IT:

■ Heat broiler and line a baking sheet with parchment. In a small bowl, mix together mustard, garlic, shallot, thyme, rosemary, and lemon juice and season with salt and pepper. Spread mixture all over salmon fillets and broil, 7 to 8 minutes.

■ Garnish with more thyme and lemon slices and serve.

MAKES 4 SERVINGS.

NUTRITION PER SERVING

570 calories

79 g protein

1 g carbohydrates (0 g fiber)

26 g fat

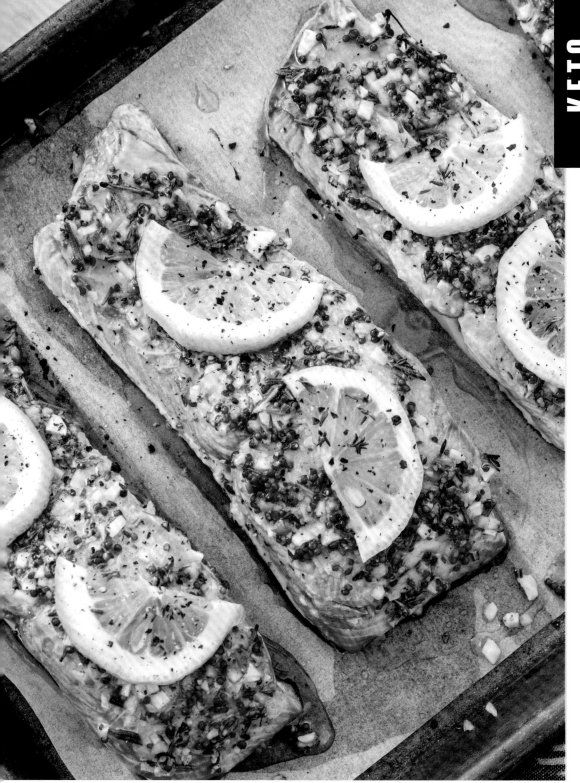

PESTO SHRIMP SKEWERS
with Cauliflower Mash

TOTAL TIME: 40 MIN

WHAT YOU'LL NEED

1   large head cauliflower, cut into small florets

Kosher salt

1   clove garlic, grated

½   cup white wine

½   cup heavy cream

¼   cup freshly grated Parmesan

3   Tbsp butter

1   lb extra-large shrimp, peeled and deveined

Bamboo skewers, soaked in water

Extra-virgin olive oil, for drizzling

Freshly ground black pepper

1   cup pesto

¼   cup chopped fresh basil for garnish

HOW TO MAKE IT

■ Fill an 8-quart pot with cool water and cauliflower florets. Cover pot and bring to a boil. Season with salt and simmer until tender, 16 to 18 minutes. (Smaller florets will speed up this step.)

■ Drain cauliflower in a colander and transfer back to pot over medium heat. Add garlic, white wine, and 1 cup water, then season with salt. Stir and cover pot, then simmer for 5 minutes. Turn off heat and add cream, then smash with a potato masher until smooth. Fold in Parmesan and butter just before serving.

■ Preheat grill or grill pan on medium-high. Thread shrimp onto skewers. Drizzle with olive oil and season with salt and pepper. Grill shrimp until lightly charred, 2 to 3 minutes on each side.

■ Serve shrimp skewers over a bed of cauliflower mash. Drizzle pesto over shrimp and garnish with fresh basil.

MAKES 4 SERVINGS.

NUTRITION PER SERVING

600 calories

29 g protein

15 g carbohydrates (5 g fiber)

45 g fat

HAM AND CHEESE EGG CUPS

TOTAL TIME: 35 MIN

WHAT YOU'LL NEED

Cooking spray, for pan

12 slices ham

1 cup shredded Cheddar

12 large eggs

Kosher salt

Freshly ground black pepper

Chopped fresh parsley,
    for garnish

HOW TO MAKE IT

■ Preheat oven to 400°F and grease a 12-cup muffin tin with cooking spray. Line each cup with a slice of ham and sprinkle with Cheddar. Crack an egg into each ham cup and season with salt and pepper.

■ Bake until eggs are cooked through, 12 to 15 minutes (depending on how runny you like your yolks).

■ Garnish with parsley and serve.

MAKES 12 SERVINGS.

NUTRITION PER SERVING

150 calories

17 g protein

1 g carbohydrates
(0 g fiber)

8 g fat

PIZZA EGGS

TOTAL TIME: 10 MIN

WHAT YOU'LL NEED

Cooking spray, for pan

1   Tbsp olive oil

2   large eggs

Kosher salt

Freshly ground black pepper

¼   cup pizza sauce, divided

¼   cup shredded mozzarella, divided

10   mini pepperoni

Freshly grated Parmesan,

for garnish

Dried oregano, for garnish

HOW TO MAKE IT

■ Spray a medium skillet over medium heat with cooking spray, then spray the inside of a mason jar lid. Place mason jar lid in the center of skillet and crack an egg inside.

■ Top with half the pizza sauce, half the cheese, and half the pepperoni. Cover with lid and cook until egg white is set and cheese is melty, 4 to 5 minutes. Repeat with remaining ingredients. Top with Parmesan and oregano, season with salt and pepper, and serve.

MAKES 2 SERVINGS.

NUTRITION PER SERVING

260 calories

13 g protein

4 g carbohydrates
(1 g fiber)

22 g fat

AVOCADO EGG IN A HOLE

TOTAL TIME: 20 MIN

WHAT YOU'LL NEED

2   avocados

2   Tbsp butter, divided

4   large eggs

Kosher salt

Freshly ground black pepper

¼   cup shredded Cheddar

2   slices cooked bacon, crumbled

2   green onions, sliced

HOW TO MAKE IT

■ Cut each avocado in half and remove pit. Lay avocado halves on their sides and carefully cut lengthwise into 2 thick slices each. Hollow out middles with a paring knife.

■ In a large, nonstick skillet over medium-low heat, melt 1 Tbsp butter. Place the 4 avocado slices into skillet and crack an egg into the center of each. Season with salt and pepper.

■ Cover skillet and cook until egg is cooked to your desired doneness, about 5 minutes for a slightly runny egg. Sprinkle cheese on top of each slice, cover with lid again and cook until the cheese is melted, 1 minute more.

■ Repeat with remaining ingredients. Garnish with bacon and green onions.

MAKES 4 SERVINGS.

NUTRITION PER SERVING

340 calories

12 g protein

10 g carbohydrates
(7 g fiber)

30 g fat

TACO BRUNCH CASSEROLE

TOTAL TIME: 50 MIN

WHAT YOU'LL NEED

1 Tbsp extra-virgin olive oil

1 lb ground beef

1 Tbsp chili powder

1 tsp ground cumin

½ tsp garlic powder

Kosher salt

Freshly ground black pepper

Cooking spray

5 large eggs

½ cup whole milk

¾ cup shredded Monterey Jack

1 cup shredded romaine lettuce

1 medium tomato, chopped

1 small avocado, halved, pitted, and diced

Sour cream, for drizzling

NUTRITION PER SERVING

506 calories

34 g protein

9 g carbohydrates (5 g fiber)

37 g fat

HOW TO MAKE IT

■ Preheat oven to 350°F. In a 10-in. ovenproof skillet over medium-high, heat oil.

■ Add ground beef and season with chili powder, cumin, garlic powder, salt, and pepper. Cook, breaking up meat with back of a wooden spoon, until beef is no longer pink, 6 to 8 minutes. Remove from heat and liberally coat the sides of the skillet with cooking spray.

■ In a medium bowl, whisk together eggs, milk, and cheese. Pour over the cooked ground beef.

■ Bake until center of eggs are set, 30 to 40 minutes.

■ Garnish with lettuce, tomatoes, avocado, and sour cream before serving.

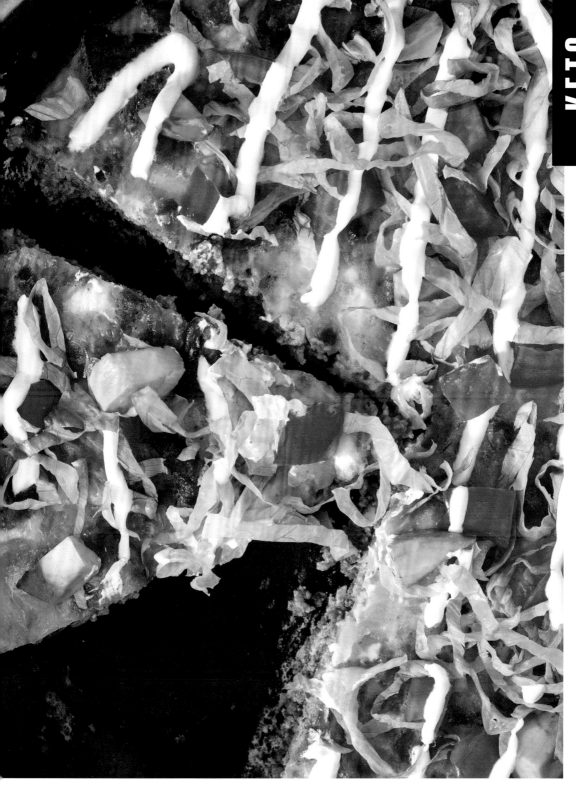

JALAPEÑO POPPER CHICKEN CASSEROLE

TOTAL TIME: 45 MIN

WHAT YOU'LL NEED

Cooking spray

1½ Tbsp extra virgin olive oil, divided

2 lb boneless, skinless chicken breasts, sliced into strips

Kosher salt

Freshly ground black pepper

1 red bell pepper, chopped

3-4 jalapeños, chopped

1 (8-oz) package cream cheese, cubed

¼ cup mayonnaise

1 cup shredded Cheddar, divided

4 slices bacon, chopped, for garnish

HOW TO MAKE IT

■ Preheat oven to 400°F. Grease an 8-in. square baking dish with cooking spray. In a large skillet over medium-high heat, heat 1 Tbsp oil. Season chicken with salt and pepper then cook until seared and no longer pink in middle, about 6 minutes per side. Remove from heat and let cool slightly before chopping into bite-size pieces.

■ In the same skillet over medium heat, heat remaining ½ Tbsp oil and cook bell pepper and jalapeños until soft, about 5 minutes. Add cream cheese, mayo, and chopped chicken, stirring until cream cheese melts. Stir in ¾ cup Cheddar and remove from heat.

■ Add chicken mixture to prepared baking dish and top with remaining ¼ cup Cheddar. Bake until cheese is melty and bubbly, 15 to 20 minutes.

■ Meanwhile, in a medium skillet over medium heat, cook bacon until crispy, about 8 minutes. Drain on a paper towel-lined plate.

■ Garnish casserole with cooked bacon pieces before serving.

MAKES 6 SERVINGS.

NUTRITION
PER SERVING

530 calories

44 g protein

5 g carbohydrates
(1 g fiber)

37 g fat

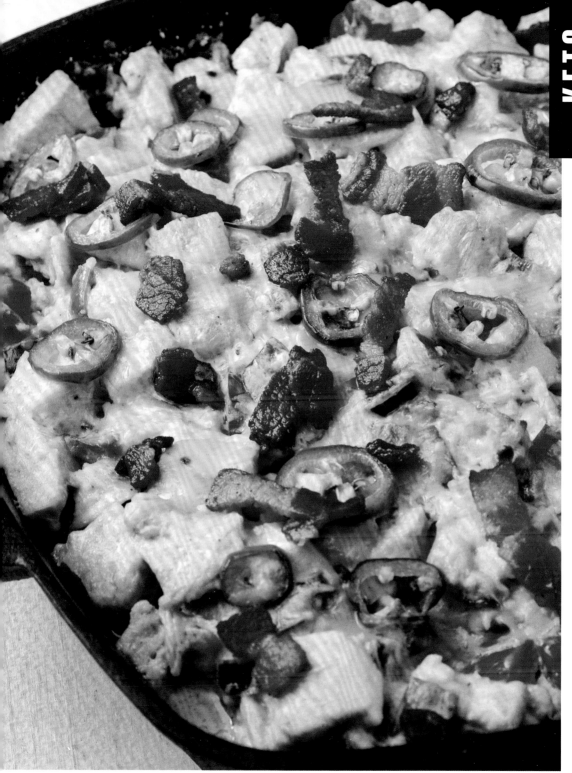

TACO CUPS

TOTAL TIME: 30 MIN

WHAT YOU'LL NEED

3½ cups shredded Cheddar

Cooking spray

1   Tbsp extra-virgin olive oil

1   onion, chopped

3   cloves garlic, minced

1   lb ground beef

1   tsp chili powder

½   tsp ground cumin

½   tsp paprika

Kosher salt

Freshly ground black pepper

Sour cream, for serving

Diced avocado, for serving

Chopped cilantro, for serving

Chopped tomatoes, for serving

HOW TO MAKE IT

■ Preheat oven to 375°F and line a large baking sheet with parchment paper. Spoon about 1 Tbsp of cheese at a time, a few inches apart. Bake until bubbly and edges are beginning to turn golden, about 6 minutes. Let cool on baking sheet for a minute.

■ Meanwhile, grease bottom of a muffin tin with cooking spray, then carefully pick up melted cheese slices and place on bottom of muffin tin. Let cool 10 minutes.

■ In a large skillet over medium, heat olive oil. Add onion and cook, stirring occasionally, until soft, about 5 minutes. Stir in garlic, then add ground beef, breaking up the meat with a wooden spoon. Cook until beef is no longer pink, about 6 minutes, then drain fat. Season with chili powder, cumin, paprika, salt, and pepper.

■ Transfer cheese cups to a serving platter. Fill with cooked ground beef, then top with sour cream, avocado, cilantro, and tomatoes.

MAKES 8 SERVINGS.

NUTRITION PER SERVING

300 calories

25 g protein

2 g carbohydrates (0 g fiber)

21 g fat

TURKEY CLUB CUPS

TOTAL TIME: 20 MIN

WHAT YOU'LL NEED

Cooking spray

12 slices roasted deli turkey

12 slices sharp Cheddar

¼ cup mayonnaise

2 Tbsp Dijon mustard

½ head iceberg lettuce, shredded

1 pint cherry tomatoes, chopped

1 avocado, halved, pitted, and chopped

8 slices bacon, cooked and chopped

HOW TO MAKE IT

■ Preheat oven to 400°F and lightly grease muffin tin with cooking spray.

■ Place a slice of turkey into each muffin cup. Add a slice of Cheddar, then bake until turkey is sturdy and cheese is melted, about 10 minutes. Let cool slightly.

■ Meanwhile, in a small bowl, mix together mayo and Dijon. Add a dollop to the bottom of each turkey cup and spread around. Fill with lettuce, cherry tomatoes, avocado, and bacon.

■ Repeat to fill cups.

MAKES 12 SERVINGS.

NUTRITION PER SERVING

230 calories

17 g protein

5 g carbohydrates (1 g fiber)

16 g fat

SLOW-COOKED BEEF STROGANOFF

TOTAL TIME: 4½ HR OR 8½ HR

WHAT YOU'LL NEED

2   lb top round beef roast, cut into 1-in. pieces

Kosher salt

Freshly ground black pepper

2   Tbsp extra virgin olive oil

1   (16-oz) package sliced mushrooms, finely chopped

½   cup low-sodium beef broth

2   cloves garlic, minced

2   tsp low-sodium soy sauce

⅓   cup sour cream

8   cups chopped cauliflower florets (from about 1 large head)

⅓   cup milk, plus more if needed

1   Tbsp butter

½   cup freshly chopped parsley, for garnish

HOW TO MAKE IT

■ Season beef with salt and pepper. In a large skillet over medium-high, heat oil. Add beef and cook until seared, 3 minutes per side.

■ Transfer beef to bowl of a large slow cooker then add mushrooms, beef broth, garlic, and soy sauce. Season with salt and pepper.

■ Cover with lid and cook until the beef is fork-tender, 4 hours on high or 8 hours on low. Turn off heat. Drain some of the liquid, if needed. Stir in sour cream and season with salt and pepper.

■ When beef is almost done, fill a large pot with 3 inches of water and add a steamer insert. Bring water to a boil over high heat then add cauliflower and cover with lid. Steam until fork tender, 12 to 15 minutes.

■ Carefully transfer cauliflower to the bowl of a food processor. Add milk and butter and season with salt and pepper. Pulse until smooth, adding a little more milk if needed.

■ Serve stroganoff over cauliflower and garnish with parsley.

MAKES 4 SERVINGS.

NUTRITION PER SERVING

390 calories

40 g protein

11 g carbohydrates (4 g fiber)

21 g fat

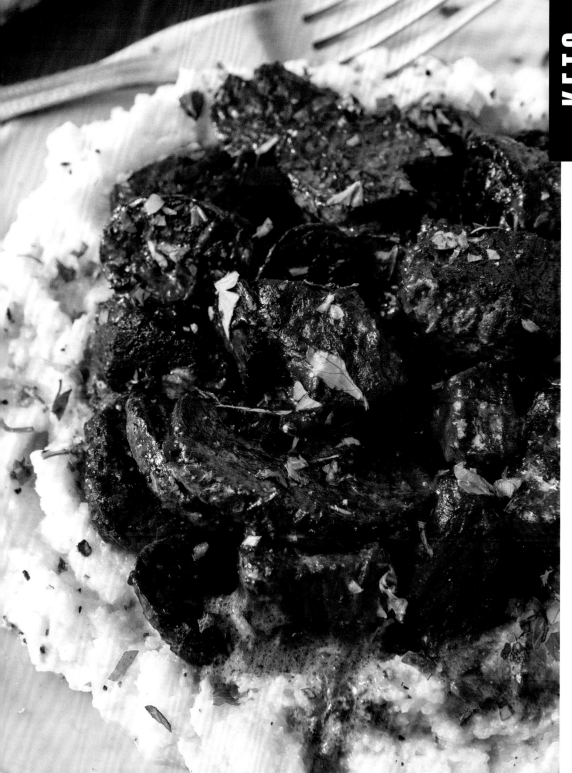

THANK YOU

FOR PURCHASING BEGINNER'S GUIDE TO IF

Boost your fitness with more from *Men's Health*.

Visit our online store and

SAVE 20% OFF YOUR NEXT PURCHASE.

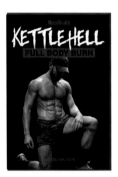 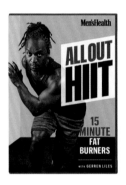 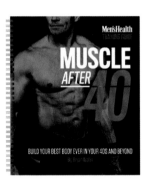

PLEASE ENJOY 20% OFF AT OUR STORE!

20%OFF

USE COUPON CODE THANKYOU20

Shop.MensHealth.com

Offer only applies to books, guides, DVDs, and new magazine subscription purchases and is not eligible on Pioneer Woman Magazine. This discount is not redeemable in combination with other promotions; additional restrictions may apply.

HEARST